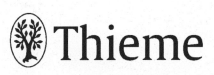

Computer Navigated and Handheld Robotic Knee Arthroplasty

An Illustrative Guide

Anoop Jhurani, MBBS, MS Orthopaedics
RORF Fellowship, Joint Replacement Surgery (HSS, NY, USA)
Director, Joint Replacement Services
Fortis Escorts Hospital
Jaipur, Rajasthan

Piyush Agarwal, MBBS, MS Orthopaedics
Consultant
Joint Replacement Services
Fortis Escorts Hospital
Jaipur, Rajasthan

Thieme
Delhi • Stuttgart • New York • Rio de Janeiro

Publishing Director: Ritu Sharma
Senior Development Editor: Dr Nidhi Srivastava
Director-Editorial Services: Rachna Sinha
Project Manager: Gaurav Prabhuzantye
Vice President-Sales and Marketing: Arun Kumar Majji
Managing Director & CEO: Ajit Kohli

Thieme Medical and Scientific Publishers Private Limited
A 12, Second Floor, Sector 2, Noida 201 301,
Uttar Pradesh, India, +911204556600
Email: customerservice@thieme.in
www.thieme.in

Cover design: © Thieme
Cover image source: © Thieme

Page make-up by RECTO Graphics, India

Printed in India

5 4 3 2

ISBN 978-93-90553-40-2

Also available as an e-book:
eISBN 978-93-90553-43-3

*Dedicated to the sacrifice of our parents and family,
to the guidance and mentorship of our teachers, camaraderie of our colleagues
and peers, questions from students and trust of our patients.*

Contents

Foreword

Advances in the field of total knee replacement surgery are occurring at an accelerating rate with improvements in implant design, materials, surgical technique, and perioperative care. Recently, computer navigation and robotics have disrupted total knee arthroplasty with an enormous influx of information. *Computer Navigated and Handheld Robotic Knee Arthroplasty: An Illustrative Guide* consolidates and integrates this rapidly evolving flow of information. It is a significant achievement to bring all these advances into one delightfully integrated text that meticulously assesses the current state of total knee arthroplasty.

    Congratulations are in order to Dr. Anoop Jhurani for bringing together a group of outstanding contributors. They have performed a wonderful job of creating presentations that are illustrative, thoughtful, and critical, thus enabling readers to benefit from their skills and knowledge. The book covers from the basics of knee arthroplasty to an in-depth discussion of navigation and robotics. We, as surgeons, will gain immeasurably from this collaboration, enabling us to serve our patients better.

Chitranjan S. Ranawat, MD
Attending Orthopedic Surgeon
Hospital for Special Surgery
New York, USA

Foreword

Knee replacement surgery is an art as much as it is a science. It has evolved over the last few decades. Different designs and different techniques have come up, each driving to perfect the results of surgery, although clinical dissatisfaction in a small number of patients still remains an issue. While the industry propagates new models every 10 to 20 years, the surgeons try to perfect their techniques. Although implants matching the patient have become available, the real goal in each individual still eludes us. What has been shown to really help is the use of computers during the surgery. It has developed over the last two decades and made its place in the techniques of surgery, helping the surgeon reproduce the desired alignment and positioning of any implant design. The robots also use computer navigation as an integral part for tracking the bones and instruments.

The author of this book, Dr. Anoop Jhurani, has been at the forefront of technology. He has visited leading international centers and brought the latest techniques to his surgical armamentarium. Not only as a surgeon but also as a teacher and leader, he has represented the fraternity at various levels. In this book, he brings in his own surgical experience together with authors of the available literature. With beautifully presented illustrations, this makes for an excellent read for the orthopaedic surgeons and trainees. A number of complex presentations are discussed. It will help readers understand the fundamentals of the knee surgery in general and use of computer navigation in difficult situations. As we know from experience, one technique cannot be applied to all the knee presentations. The tips provided in the book will help surgeons navigate through a complex procedure, adding to the patient outcomes and experience. Knowledge combined with experience brings out the best in a surgeon. This book will elevate the readers with knowledge as well as the collective wisdom of the authors, thus helping them to produce the best outcomes for their patients.

Kamal Deep, MBBS, DO, MS, DNB, FRCS, MCh Orth, FRCS Orth
CEO
Healthcare Education Delivery Ltd.
Consultant Orthopaedic Surgeon
Glasgow, United Kingdom;
Executive Member
CAOS UK (The British Society for Computer Assisted Orthopaedic Surgery) and CAOS International

Preface

The outcomes of partial and total knee arthroplasty continue to evolve and improve. The main factors contributing to enhanced function after knee arthroplasty are better understanding of soft tissue behavior, innovative implant design, materials, and use of technology.

Technologies like computer navigation and robotics help in objective assessment and analysis of deformity and soft tissue behavior. This in turn guides the bone resection to achieve the desired correction with optimal soft tissue release. We have used computer-assisted and handheld robotics to manage all routine and complex cases for nearly a decade now. Through careful observation and recording of data, we have been able to introduce some new concepts and challenge old ones.

Our main interest has been to study the correlation and interplay of coronal and sagittal plane deformity and predict the correction of sagittal plane when coronal deformity is corrected. Similarly, through concerted work and efforts we have outlined some key concepts for challenging cases of extra-articular deformities, implants in situ, and polyarticular presentations.

The aim of writing this book is to present new findings and ideas in a clear and concise manner so that the reader can unlearn outdated concepts and learn fresh ones. We think that this illustrative guide will be useful to the trainee and the trainer alike.

This book is presented in a point-wise format citing case examples and providing navigation/robotic screenshots for easy understanding and interpretation. Various aspects of our ideas are highlighted in *Principles, Pearls, Pitfalls*, and *Points to Remember* sections in each chapter to bring forth key concepts and reiterate important tips.

We sincerely hope that this book will be a valuable asset in your library.

Anoop Jhurani, MBBS, MS Orthopaedics
Piyush Agarwal, MBBS, MS Orthopaedics

Contributors

Anoop Jhurani, MBBS, MS Orthopaedics
RORF Fellowship, Joint Replacement Surgery (HSS, NY, USA)
Director, Joint Replacement Services
Fortis Escorts Hospital
Jaipur, Rajasthan

Piyush Agarwal, MBBS, MS Orthopaedics
Consultant
Joint Replacement Services
Fortis Escorts Hospital
Jaipur, Rajasthan

Kunal Aneja, MBBS, MS, DNB, MCh (UK)
Managing Director and Chief Orthopaedic Surgeon
Naveda Healthcare Centres
New Delhi, Delhi

Mukesh Aswal, MBBS, MS Orthopaedics
Associate Consultant
Joint Replacement Services
Fortis Escorts Hospital
Jaipur, Rajasthan

Role of Computer Navigation in Knee Arthroplasty

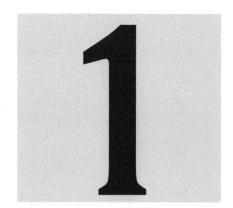

Anoop Jhurani and Piyush Agarwal

Introduction

- The function and survivorship of total knee arthroplasty (TKA) depends on implant positioning, overall limb alignment, and soft tissue balance.[1]
- Malalignment and ligament imbalance may cause polyethylene wear and early implant loosening, thereby decreasing the survivorship of a replaced knee.[2]
- Attaining overall coronal mechanical alignment of limb within ±3 degrees of varus/valgus and 0 to 5 degrees of flexion has proved to be important predictor of TKA function and longevity.[3]
- Computer assisted surgery (CAS) gives objective quantification of coronal/sagittal deformity and helps assess unique soft tissue behavior of every knee.
- This aids in optimizing bone resection and soft tissue releases to achieve ideal limb alignment and ligament balance.

Advantages of Computer Navigation

Better Accuracy

- As opposed to the conventional method, CAS has shown to produce better accuracy of bony cuts which results in improved overall limb alignment.[1] Based on the deformity in coronal and sagittal planes, bony cuts can be planned with respect to thickness, flexion/extension, and varus/valgus.
- With CAS, there is reduction in incidence of prosthesis malpositioning.[2]
- It also leads to decreased rate of revision surgery due to accurate prosthesis positioning and optimal alignment (**Fig. 1.1** and **Fig. 1.2**).[3,4]
- Studies have shown that computer navigation eliminates alignment "outliers." Experienced surgeons, using conventional alignment systems, can accurately align the

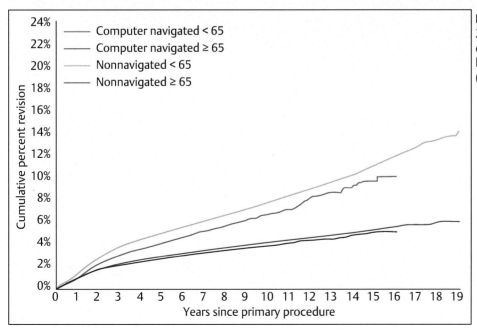

Fig. 1.1 Australian Registry Report 2020. Cumulative percent revision of primary total knee replacement by computer navigation and age (primary diagnosis OA).

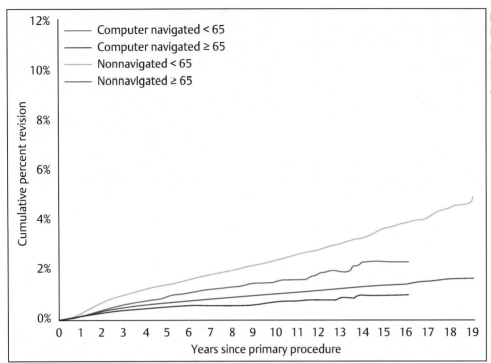

Fig. 1.2 Australian Registry Report 2020. Cumulative percent revision for loosening of primary total knee replacement by computer navigation and age (primary diagnosis OA).

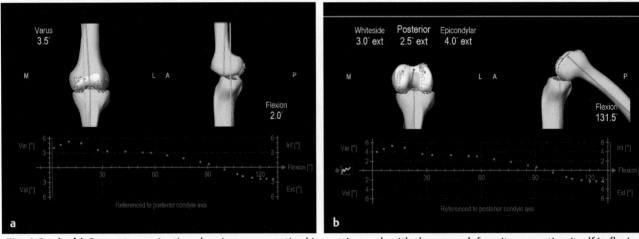

Fig. 1.3 **(a, b)** Computer navigation showing preoperative kinematic graph with the varus deformity correcting itself in flexion.

knee in over 90 to 95% of cases. However, studies show that in as many as 5 to 10% of surgeries, postoperative knee alignment can be less than ideal. The patients in this 5 to 10% group are considered "outliers." It is believed that computer navigation's accuracy can assist the surgeon in shrinking the percentage of alignment outliers.[5]

- Published literature illustrates that the bony cuts are reproducible to a greater extent when guided by computer navigation as compared to conventional alignment systems, thus minimizing the surgical error.[6]

- Titration of soft tissue release: In computer-assisted navigation, software reveals the knee deformity throughout the range of motion. In the majority of the patients

with varus deformity of the knee, the deformity corrects itself when the knee is flexed. Hence, minimal soft tissue release of anteriomedial structures is required to achieve harmonious soft tissue balance (**Fig. 1.3**).

- Accurate mediolateral gap balancing: Navigation accurately reveals any mediolateral imbalance with a trial prosthesis, thus enabling the surgeon to fine-tune ligament balance with minimal soft tissue releases. This reduces the chances of instability at any point in the arc of motion (**Fig. 1.4**).[7]

- Early rehabilitation and shorter hospital stay are required after CAS TKA due to good limb alignment and accurate gap balancing.[1]

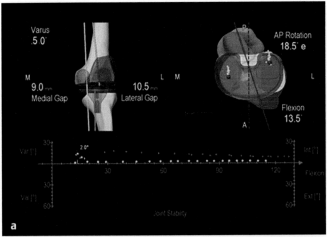
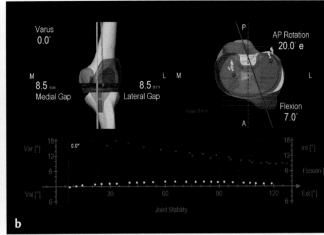

Fig. 1.4   (a, b) Computer navigation showing coronal and sagittal alignment in extension. Soft tissue releases and bone cuts can be rationalized for complete correction of the deformity.

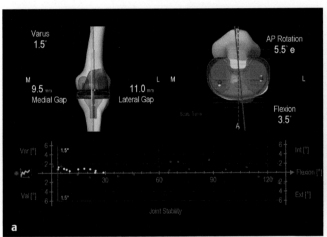
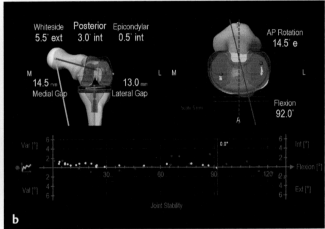

Fig. 1.5   (a, b) Computer navigation showing soft tissue balance in extension and 90-degree flexion.

- In conventional TKR surgery, the knee ligaments are balanced chiefly by the surgeon's ability to "feel" and determine if the ligaments are appropriately taut. Although experienced surgeons can achieve excellent knee balance in the majority of the cases, reproducibility is difficult and results are subjective. With computer navigation, ligament balancing can potentially be quantified to the nearest millimeter of ligament laxity or tautness.[8] As computer navigation software improves, the surgeon's ability to balance the ligaments of the knee would become more precise. This, ultimately, may prove to be computer navigation's greatest advantage over conventional surgery (**Fig. 1.5**).
- Accurate gap balancing helps in restoring the height of the joint line and the posterior offset.[9]

Minimally Invasive Surgery

- The usage of computer navigation complements the minimally invasive surgical techniques for TKA. Thus, smaller incisions with decreased soft tissue disruption result in reduced pain and accelerated recovery postoperatively.
- Although blind insertion of pins may violate this benefit, usage of stab incision and sleeves can protect the surrounding soft tissues. This protects the quadriceps muscle and tendon during surgery.[10]

Dynamic Assessment of Deformity

- Utilizing CAS, surgeons can assess the deformity at any angle of flexion, whereas in conventional total knee replacement (TKR), deformity is measured only in knee extension. This is possible due to the intraoperative range of motion (ROM) kinematic analysis provided by computer navigation (**Fig. 1.6**).[2]
- Careful analysis of the kinematic graph helps in planning the bony cuts and making the necessary adjustments before execution.
- The kinematic graph also helps in titrating the soft tissue release in cases with biplanar deformity.[1]

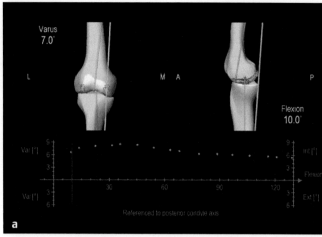 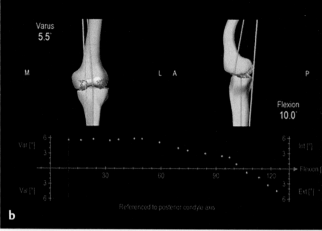

Fig. 1.6 (a, b) Different kinematics for similar deformity in two different patients demonstrating uncorrectable varus with knee flexion in first case and varus fully correcting with knee flexion in second case (Pink dots).

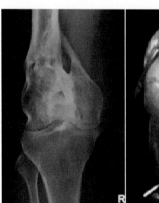 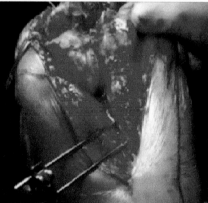 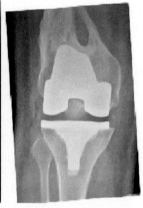

Fig. 1.7 Computer-navigated total knee replacement (TKR) in malunited distal femur fracture.

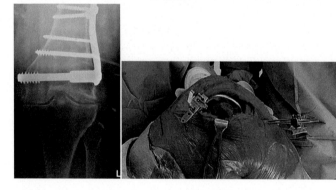 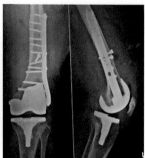

Fig. 1.8 Computer-navigated total knee replacement (TKR) in united supracondylar femur fracture with dynamic compression screw (DCS) in situ.

Advantageous in Complicated Cases

- Conventional alignment systems can be difficult or impossible to use if there is a significant extra-articular deformity in the femur or tibia. This is due to the requirement of an unobstructed femoral and tibial canal for the intramedullary (IM) systems (**Fig. 1.7**).[11]
- Conventional TKR is difficult to execute in cases with implants in the medullary canal from previous trauma surgery. CAS helps in solving these complex problems without removal of previous implants and obviating the need for additional incisions/surgery. This is possible as CAS bypasses the IM implants and uses external landmarks to achieve proper component and limb alignment (**Fig. 1.8**).[12]
- Thus, patients with an extra-articular bony deformity or retained hardware around the knee are ideal candidates for utilizing computer navigation.

Teaching Tool

- The most important and under-rated advantage of navigation is documentation. It not only helps in quantifying the deformity but also records the patient's preoperative, intraoperative, and postoperative knee kinematics This information can be utilized for clinical and scientific documentation, which is useful for performing research and improving techniques.[13]
- It is an excellent teaching tool wherein the trainee can be taught the behavior of a particular knee by analyzing the consequence of every surgical step during the procedure.[13]

Systemic Advantages

- Computer navigation guidance eliminates the requirement for an alignment rod to be placed inside the IM canal of the femur (**Fig. 1.9**).
- Usage of computer navigation results in lower plasma D-Dimer levels in comparison to patients undergoing TKA with the conventional technique. This results in a decreased risk of pulmonary thromboembolism events postoperatively.[14]
- Elimination of the need to open the IM canal in navigation or robotic-assisted surgery results in decreased blood loss. This translates to a decreased requirement of blood transfusion for the patient.[15]
- Decreased rate of pulmonary embolism due to extramedullary instrumentation results in a lowered risk of acute cerebrovascular and/or cardiac events, especially in simultaneous bilateral TKA.[16]

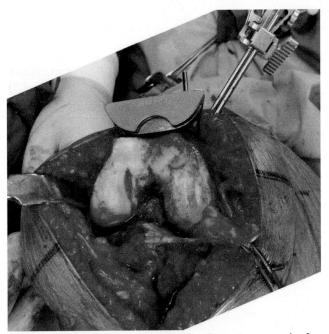

Fig. 1.9 Computer navigation eliminates need for intramedullary hole in femur.

Disadvantages and Complications

- Use of computer navigation is still not widely accepted among arthroplasty surgeons.
- Apprehension of increased tourniquet time and insertion of additional pins is an impeding factor.
- Computer navigation and robotics have their own set of pitfalls and complications.
- With better understanding of the technology, one can overcome the potential complications and use the technology to achieve improved surgical outcomes.[17]
- Robotics in arthroplasty is still an emerging technology. It shares the same complications as associated with computer navigation, with an additional drawback of specificity.
- The commercially available robots currently available are specific to a particular company or prosthesis. This lack of versatility may discourage surgeon from using a particular technology.[18]

Potential Disadvantages of Navigation

Increased Operative Time

- The increase in operating time ranges from 10 to 30 minutes, depending upon the surgeon's experience in using CAS for TKA.[1]
- This increased operating time is usually consumed during verification of cuts, nondetection of the array by the camera unit, loosening of pin or array, etc.
- However, studies have shown that as experience is gained, learning curve is negotiated and operative time decreases significantly.[2]

Pearls

With time, the surgeon can predict the best position for camera unit and arrays attached to the bones; this prevents nondetection of trackers by camera unit intraoperatively.

- Prolonged tourniquet use may lead to increased tourniquet time. This may result in complications such as increased postoperative pain, embolism, increased blood loss, delayed wound healing, etc.[19]

Pearls

- The authors avoid using a tourniquet during surgery. A combination of improved surgical technique, better hemostasis, and hypotensive anesthesia provides a bloodless operating field.
- *One can minimize the usage of a tourniquet* by inflating it only during cementation of the prosthesis.

Additional Incisions Required for Array Fixation

Whenever possible, the authors prefer to keep the pin within the skin incision of TKA. In an anatomically small knee and for minimally invasive surgical technique, the surgeon can give stab incisions with the number 11 surgical blade for pin insertion.

Pearls

Sleeves should be utilized while inserting the pins blindly through the stab incisions to avoid causing iatrogenic fractures and potential damage to the quadriceps muscle (**Fig. 1.10**).

Periprosthetic Fractures

- The pin site can be a potential stress riser, which can lead to of periprosthetic fractures through pin sites (**Fig. 1.11**).
- Pinholes alter the biomechanical strength of the bone, especially femur. They can decrease the bending strength and energy-absorbing characteristics of the bone by up to 40%.[20]
- Most of the periprosthetic fractures occur within 3 months of surgery (**Fig. 1.12**).[21]
- The potential risk factors which predispose the bone to periprosthetic fractures are:
  - Bicortical drilling.
  - Usage of thick Schanz screws.
  - Anterior placement of pins in diaphyseal bone.
  - Bending of pins by tracker clamping system.
  - Thermal necrosis caused by high-speed drilling.
  - Osteoporotic bone.
  - Repeated attempts at pin placement.
  - Multiple repeated bony cuts along with pinholes concentrated over a small area, especially medial femoral condyle, predispose to periprosthetic fracture on weight bearing.
- The development of a periprosthetic fracture requires readmission and revision surgery in the majority of the cases, contributing to increased morbidity.
- Thomas et al documented fracture incidence of 1.38% through the femoral pin tracker site.[22]
- To reduce the incidence of periprosthetic fractures, the authors prefer:
  - Usage of two 3-mm Schanz screws.
  - Unicortical purchase instead of bicortical drilling.

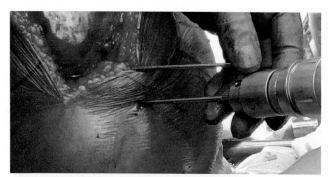

Fig. 1.10 Additional incision for Schanz pin.

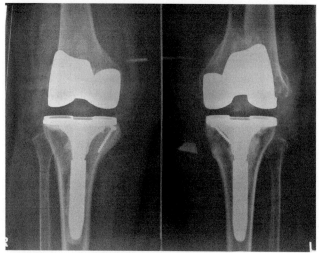

Fig. 1.11 Postoperative X-ray showing a periprosthetic fracture in the distal femur at the pin tract site.

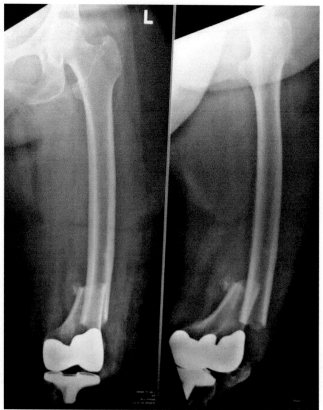

Fig. 1.12 Postoperative X-ray showing periprosthetic fracture in femur from proximal pin tract site.

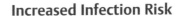

- The pin insertion into the metadiaphyseal cancellous region of the bone, which has greater healing potential and broader morphology, providing greater area of purchase.
- The pins should be placed as perpendicular to the cortex as possible to prevent the stress riser effect.
- Protection sleeves with low-speed and high-torque drills should be used for pin placement.

Pearls

At the end of the procedure, the authors prefer to plug the pinholes with a conical piece of bone shaped from medial sclerotic part of tibial cut. These triangular bony pieces act as autologous bone grafts, promoting faster healing, and plugging the pinholes prevents further blood loss (**Fig. 1.13** and **Fig. 1.14**).

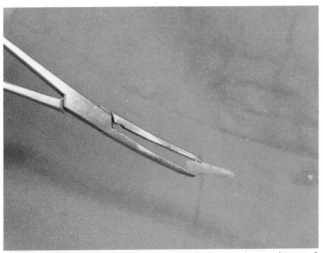

Fig. 1.13　Triangular bone plugs made from sclerotic bone of distal femur or proximal tibia cut.

Increased Infection Risk

- Increased surgical time theoretically increases the risk of infection due to the surgical wound being open for a longer duration.[23]
- However, the available literature has not revealed a greater infection rate in computer navigation surgeries (presumably due to the relatively modest increase in surgical time).[24]
- Surgeons experienced in the usage of computer navigation systems may limit the increase in the duration of the surgical procedure by 10 minutes or less. With greater advancement in artificial intelligence and machine-based learning, along with improvement in computer navigation and robotics systems, the time difference between navigation and conventional procedures will diminish.[25]
- Superficial pin site infections: Pin site complications like pin site infections are rarely encountered and the reported incidence is less than 1%.[26]

Increased Cost

- The chief disadvantage of using computer navigation is the increased cost associated with it.
- There is a considerable upfront capital expense to the hospital to purchase and maintain computer navigation systems.
- Insurance companies and Medicare do not increase the reimbursement for surgeries utilizing computer navigation, hence forcing the hospitals to absorb the additional expense.
- Many leading joint replacement hospitals have acquired navigation systems to provide the cutting-edge technology and provide best available care to their patients.
- At many centers, the additional cost of using technology is not passed on to the patients undergoing the surgery.
- Studies have shown that the usage of computer navigation has decreased the rate of revision in the long term.[27]

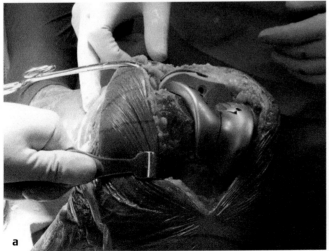
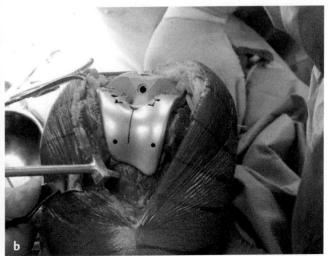

Fig. 1.14　**(a, b)** These bony plugs can be inserted into the pinholes with the help of bone punch and mallet.

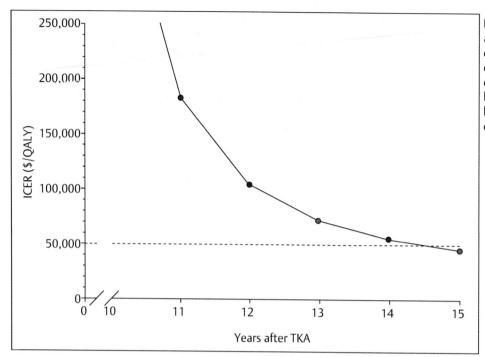

Fig. 1.15 One-way sensitivity analysis of incremental cost effectiveness ratio (ICER) of computer-assisted surgery compared with mechanical guides by years of follow-up after total knee arthroplasty (TKA). QALY, quality-adjusted life-year.

Pearls

If the cost of revision surgery due to malalignment of the prosthesis is considered, computer navigation proves to be cost-effective or cost-saving from a long-term perspective (**Fig. 1.15**).[28]

Learning Curve

- To master a new technique or technology, a learning curve needs to be negotiated.[29]
- The learning curve associated with CAS or RAS creates a sense of apprehension among the arthroplasty surgeons, making them reluctant to adopt it for their routine clinical practice.
- The surgeons may find it technically demanding or time-consuming for a regular case.
- Computer navigation provides constant visual and numerical feedback throughout the surgery (concurrent extrinsic feedback), which enables the surgeon to shorten the learning curve associated with it.[29]
- The surgeon becomes more used to the workflow of the navigation screen over time.
- Besides, after familiarizing oneself with computer planning and graphics, the surgeon can modify his surgical practice and technique, like the appropriate usage of instruments, keeping the limb in ideal position, etc. This decreases the challenges encountered while operating and translates to reduced operating time.
- Appropriate clinical workshops, cadaveric training, and working with experienced navigation/ robotic surgeons for hands-on experience can be inculcated as part of the surgical training to improve the skill over time.

Pearls

Literature suggests that a new surgeon can perform a navigated TKA with the same efficiency and precision as the experienced surgeon after first 50 cases using computer navigation.[30]

Pin Breakage/Loosening

- This complication although rare has been well documented in the literature and could potentially jeopardize the entire workflow intraoperatively.

Pearls

To prevent this complication:
- Array clamps should be duly checked before starting the registration process.
- In cases with a thin cortex or where the bony purchase is doubtful, it is advisable to place the pins more distally in the supracondylar region of the femur for better purchase.
- Pins and arrays should be handled with care intraoperatively and caution exercised to avoid hitting them with a saw blade or any other instrument.
- The authors prefer to remove the femoral and tibial array while executing the bony cuts or during trial insertion to avoid any damage. The arrays are placed over clamps only during the steps of registration and verification.

- Potential reasons which result in pin breakage or loosening intraoperatively are:
  – Loose pins at the time of insertion.

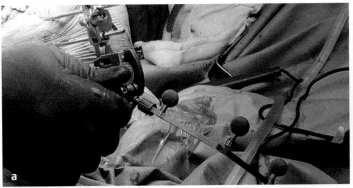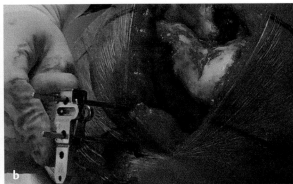

Fig. 1.16   (a, b) Array and pin clamps should be tightened before registration.

- Not tightening the array clamps (**Fig. 1.16**).
- Osteoporotic bone.
- Wrong technique of pin insertion.
- The pins may loosen up when they are hit by a saw blade or any other surgical instrument.

Referencing Error by the Surgeon

- The anatomical landmarks are selected by the surgeon during the registration process.
- Bony landmarks can be registered inaccurately in obese patients or excessively deformed knees. This leads to wrong data interpretation and incorrect bony cuts, resulting in malaligned components.[31]

Pearls

- Adequate time should be given for the registration process, as the subsequent procedure depends completely on it.
- Bony landmarks like medial malleolus should be felt before doing registration, especially in obese patients.
- With the passage of time and gaining surgical experience, one can overcome this limitation.

Increased Pain

- Due to prolonged operative and tourniquet time, patients may experience increased pain postoperatively.
- The pinholes, which act as stress risers, can also lead to increased thigh pain.

Pearls

- Limit/avoid usage of the tourniquet.
- A cocktail injection administered locally may decrease the acute pain related to increased operative duration and potential quadriceps damage.
- The surgeon should be vigilant for prolonged/severe localized thigh pain as it may be indicative of impending periprosthetic fracture.[32]

References

1. Bae DK, Song SJ, Yoon KH, Noh JH, Lee CH. Intraoperative assessment of resected condyle thickness in total knee arthroplasty. Knee Surg Sports Traumatol Arthrosc 2012;20(10):2039–2046

2. Deep K, Shankar S, Mahendra A. Computer assisted navigation in total knee and hip arthroplasty. SICOT J 2017;3:50

3. Schnurr C, Güdden I, Eysel P, König DP. Influence of computer navigation on TKA revision rates. Int Orthop 2012;36(11): 2255–2260

4. NJRRA. (2016) Australian National Joint Registry Annual Report 2016, https://aoanjrr.sahmri.com/annual-reports-2016

5. Kim SJ, MacDonald M, Hernandez J, Wixson RL. Computer assisted navigation in total knee arthroplasty: improved coronal alignment. J Arthroplasty 2005; 20(7, Suppl 3):123–131

6. Mullaji A, Sharma A, Marawar S, Kanna R. Quantification of effect of sequential posteromedial release on flexion and extension gaps: a computer-assisted study in cadaveric knees. J Arthroplasty 2009;24(5):795–805

7. Lee DH, Park JH, Song DI, Padhy D, Jeong WK, Han SB. Accuracy of soft tissue balancing in TKA: comparison between navigation-assisted gap balancing and conventional measured resection. Knee Surg Sports Traumatol Arthrosc 2010;18(3):381–387

8. Stiehl JB, Heck DA. How precise is computer-navigated gap assessment in TKA? Clin Orthop Relat Res 2015;473(1):115–118

9. Ee G, Pang HN, Chong HZ, Tan MH, et al. Computer navigation improves accuracy of joint line restoration in total knee arthroplasty. Orthop Proc 2012;94-B SUPP_XLIV:30–30

10. Stulberg SD, Yaffe MA, Koo SS. Computer-assisted surgery versus manual total knee arthroplasty: a case-controlled study. J Bone Joint Surg Am 2006;88(Suppl 4):47–54

11. Rajgopal A, Vasdev A, Dahiya V, Tyagi VC, Gupta H. Total knee arthroplasty in extra articular deformities: a series of 36 knees. Indian J Orthop 2013;47(1):35–39

12. Tigani D, Masetti G, Sabbioni G, Ben Ayad R, Filanti M, Fosco M. Computer-assisted surgery as indication of choice: total knee arthroplasty in case of retained hardware or extra-articular deformity. Int Orthop 2012;36(7):1379–1385

13. Beal MD, Delagramaticas D, Fitz D. Improving outcomes in total knee arthroplasty—do navigation or customized implants have a role? J Orthop Surg Res 2016;11(1):60

14. Siu K-K, Wu K-T, Ko J-Y, et al. Effects of computer-assisted navigation versus the conventional technique for total knee arthroplasty on levels of plasma thrombotic markers: a prospective study. Biomed Eng Online 2019;18(1):99

15. Schnurr C, Csécsei G, Eysel P, König DP. The effect of computer navigation on blood loss and transfusion rate in TKA. Orthopedics 2010;33(7):474

16. Ooi LH, Lo NN, Yeo SJ, Ong BC, Ding ZP, Lefi A. Does computer-assisted surgical navigation total knee arthroplasty reduce venous thromboembolism compared with conventional total knee arthroplasty? Singapore Med J 2008;49(8):610–614

17. Suero EM, Lueke U, Stuebig T, Hawi N, Krettek C, Liodakis E. Computer navigation for total knee arthroplasty achieves better postoperative alignment compared to conventional and patient-specific instrumentation in a low-volume setting. Orthop Traumatol Surg Res 2018;104(7):971–975

18. Netravali NA, Shen F, Park Y, Bargar WL. A perspective on robotic assistance for knee arthroplasty. Adv Orthop 2013;2013:970703

19. Zhang W, Li N, Chen S, Tan Y, Al-Aidaros M, Chen L. The effects of a tourniquet used in total knee arthroplasty: a meta-analysis. J Orthop Surg Res 2014;9(1):13

20. Bonutti P, Dethmers D, Stiehl JB. Case report: femoral shaft fracture resulting from femoral tracker placement in navigated TKA. Clin Orthop Relat Res 2008;466(6):1499–1502

21. Yoo JD, Kim NK. Periprosthetic fractures following total knee arthroplasty. Knee Surg Relat Res 2015;27(1):1–9

22. Thomas A, Pemmaraju G, Nagra G, Bassett J, Deshpande S. Complications resulting from tracker pin-sites in computer navigated knee replacement surgery. Acta Orthop Belg 2015;81(4):708–712

23. Peersman G, Laskin R, Davis J, Peterson MG, Richart T. Prolonged operative time correlates with increased infection rate after total knee arthroplasty. HSS J 2006;2(1):70–72

24. Kuo S-J, Hsu H-C, Wang C-J, et al. Effects of computer-assisted navigation versus conventional total knee arthroplasty on the levels of inflammation markers: A prospective study. PLoS One 2018;13(5):e0197097

25. Jenny J-Y, Picard F. Learning navigation: learning with navigation. A review. SICOT J 2017;3:39

26. Owens RF Jr, Swank ML. Low incidence of postoperative complications due to pin placement in computer-navigated total knee arthroplasty. J Arthroplasty 2010;25(7):1096–1098

27. de Steiger RN, Liu YL, Graves SE. Computer navigation for total knee arthroplasty reduces revision rate for patients less than sixty-five years of age. J Bone Joint Surg Am 2015;97(8):635–642

28. Novak EJ, Silverstein MD, Bozic KJ. The cost-effectiveness of computer-assisted navigation in total knee arthroplasty. J Bone Joint Surg Am 2007;89(11):2389–2397

29. Smith BRK, Deakin AH, Baines J, Picard F. Computer navigated total knee arthroplasty: the learning curve. Comput Aided Surg 2010;15(1-3):40–48

30. Gofton W, Dubrowski A, Tabloie F, Backstein D. The effect of computer navigation on trainee learning of surgical skills. J Bone Joint Surg Am 2007;89(12):2819–2827

31. Brin YS, Livshetz I, Antoniou J, Greenberg-Dotan S, Zukor DJ. Precise landmarking in computer assisted total knee arthroplasty is critical to final alignment. J Orthop Res 2010;28(10):1355–1359

32. McGraw P, Kumar A. Periprosthetic fractures of the femur after total knee arthroplasty. J Orthop Traumatol 2010;11(3):135–141

Setting of Navigation in Operating Room, Data Acquisition, and Interpretation

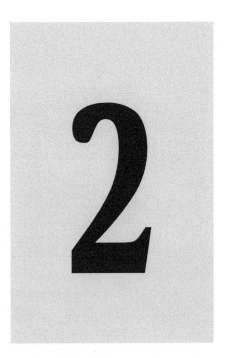

Anoop Jhurani, Piyush Agarwal, and Kunal Aneja

Components of Computer Navigation

The navigation system comprises of computer platform, tracking system, and tracker/marker.

Computer Platform

- A computer with an in-built navigation software is given various inputs from the surgical field like the center of the femoral head, surface landmarks of the distal femur, and proximal tibia with the center of the ankle joint.[1]
- It further interprets the obtained data and morphs a model of femur and tibia that best fits to a particular patient's anatomy (**Fig. 2.1**).

Tracking Systems

The tracking system is composed of an optical camera, ultrasound probe, electromagnetic coil, electromagnetic pulse, or ultrasonic waves that originate from trackers.[2]

Trackers/Markers

Markers can be of two types:
- *Active markers*: Emits light from a bulb and has a battery or wire as a power source.
- *Passive markers*: Reflects infrared (IR) light (**Fig. 2.2**).

Preoperative Preparation

- The preparation for a navigated total knee replacement should include the *setup of a computer camera unit in the operation room* so that it does not interfere with the operative procedure.
- The *camera unit* should be placed either at the opposite side of the knee being operated or at the foot end of the table, so that both the femoral and tibial arrays are detectable in the entire range of motion.
- The computer monitor unit must be *clearly visible to the operating surgeon* without any obstruction (**Fig. 2.3**).
- The surgeon can choose one of the femoral rotation references among the three available ones (**Fig. 2.4**).
- A choice can be made to navigate to the planned resections or bone references.
- The choice to enable kinematic analysis and femoral bow can also be made. Usually kinematic analysis is chosen as it gives a complete picture of knee deformity and its behavior throughout the range of motion.
- The surgeon can choose the workflow sequence planned during the procedure (**Fig. 2.5**).
- A choice has to be made among the gap balanced vs. measured resection approach.
- The registration can be either *standard or split*, with an option for *express registration*.

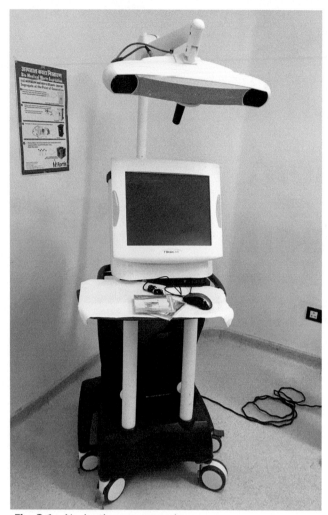

Fig. 2.1 Navigation camera unit.

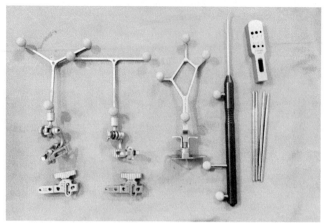

Fig. 2.2 This image shows the instruments used for computer navigation which include (left to right): Y-shape femoral array, T-shaped tibial array, two clamps, four points cutting array, pointer, four Schanz screws of 3.2 mm size, screw clamp for screw placement.

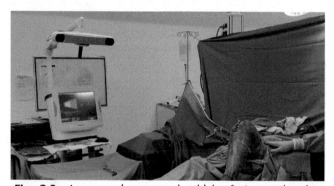

Fig. 2.3 Arrays and camera should be facing each other without any obstacle.

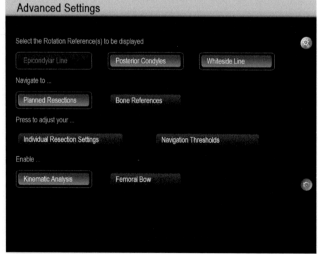

Fig. 2.4 Advanced settings for femoral rotation and balancing.

Fig. 2.5 Advanced settings for workflow sequence and planning approach.

Pearls

The authors prefer a femur first approach because tibia first requires forceful anterior dislocation of tibia, excessive soft issue releases and manipulation.

- *The femoral rotation* can be chosen with reference to the epicondylar axis, posterior condylar axis, or Whiteside line (**Fig. 2.6**).
- *Transepicondylar axis:*
  - The axis connecting the medial and lateral epicondyles.
  - There is high possibility for inter- and intraobserver variability due to inconsistency in locating and marking the epicondyles.
- *Whiteside line:*
  - The line connecting the center of the intercondylar notch and deepest point of the trochlear groove.
  - Intercondylar osteophytes can make its identification difficult.
  - It is less reliable than posterior condyles.

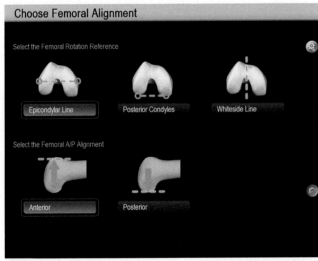

Fig. 2.6 Setting for femoral rotation reference and anteroposterior (AP) alignment.

- *Posterior condylar axis:*
  - Posterior condyle referencing is the most reliable among these as it is clearly identifiable.
  - Posterior condyle wear should be carefully evaluated (usually the medial condyle in a varus knee and the lateral condyle in a valgus knee) to prevent malrotation of femoral component.
- The *femoral A/P alignment* can be chosen to be anterior or posterior referencing as per the surgeon's preference (**Table 2.1**).

Pearls

- The authors prefer posterior condylar line as a reference to decide the rotation of the femoral component. It is cross-checked with interepicondylar axis and Whiteside line.
- The authors prefer anterior referencing over posterior referencing as there is flexibility to downsize the femoral component with ease without overstuffing the anterior offset or notching the anterior femoral cortex.

Navigation for Total Knee Replacement

- Image free navigation is the most commonly used navigation system.
- The authors use the image-free computer navigation system of *Brain Lab.*
- The use of navigation in total knee replacement involves the following *basic steps*, which are described in detail below:
  - Fixation of arrays.
  - Registration.
  - Navigation cutting blocks.
  - Verification of cuts.
  - Gap balancing.
  - Final alignment.

Table 2.1 Anterior referencing vs. posterior referencing

Parameters	Anterior referencing	Posterior referencing
Reference	Anterior femoral cortex	Posterior femoral condyle
Downsizing femoral component	Easier	Difficult
Anterior femoral notching	Reduced risk	Increased risk
Chances of flexion instability	Increased due to increased posterior condylar bone resection.	Decreased since femoral posterior offset is maintained
Risk of overstuffing anterior offset	Reduced	Increased
If femur size in between	Smaller femoral component	Larger femoral component

Fixation of Arrays

- After initial exposure, the femoral and tibial arrays are attached to the distal third of the femur and proximal third of the tibia (**Fig. 2.7**).
- These arrays are fixed to the bone using the unicortical placement of two Shanz screws on both femur and tibia.
- It is important to place the pins accurately or else the registration process may fail.
- The optimum diameter for the screws is selected, as a smaller diameter may result in loosening during surgery, while a larger diameter screw may result in a big hole, predisposing to fracture.
- Two screws of 3 mm diameter each are preferred over one 5-mm bicortical screw, to avoid the incidence of periprosthetic fractures.[1]
- It is advisable to use two screws rather than one, as a single pin has higher chances of loosening.[1]
- These Shanz screws may be placed within the surgical wound or outside it, but they should be placed in such a manner, that they do not interfere with the positioning of cutting guides or prostheses (**Fig. 2.8** to **Fig. 2.10**).

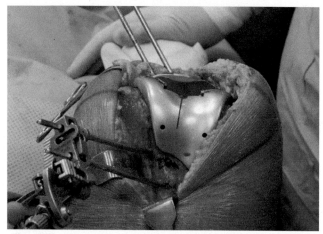

Fig. 2.7 Demonstrating the proper placement of Schanz screws in the femur, within the surgical wound and away from prosthesis.

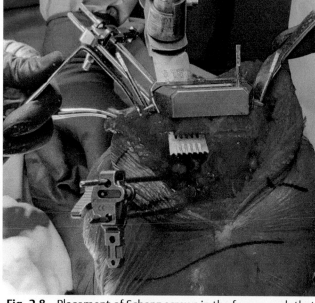

Fig. 2.8 Placement of Schanz screws in the femur, such that they do not interfere with the femoral jig placement.

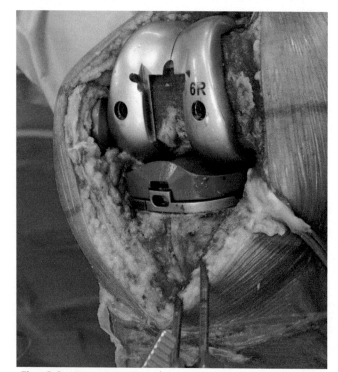

Fig. 2.9 Demonstrating the proper placement of Schanz screws in the Tibia, away from the placement of jig and the trial components.

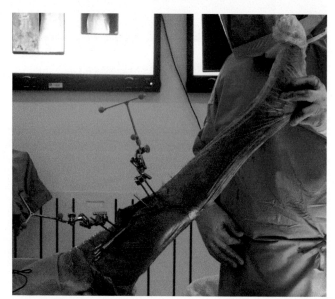

Fig. 2.10 The arrays are placed at a divergent angle of 45 degrees, so that they don't touch each other when the knee is extended.

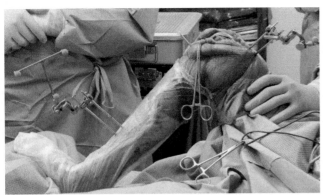

Fig. 2.11 The Schanz screws can be placed in the diaphyseal region if an intramedullary stem is planned.

- Placing the pins in the diaphyseal region of femur and tibia increases the chances of periprosthetic fractures (**Fig. 2.11** and **Fig. 2.12**).

Pitfalls

It is advised that the surgeon should only engage the second cortex and not pass the pin through it.

- If the pins are placed too distally, they may impinge with the distal cutting femoral jig placement or the femoral trial component.
- The distal tibial pin is fixed on the medial side, at the level of tibial tuberosity above the insertion of pes anserinus, while the proximal pin is placed further medially so that neither of the pins interferes with the placement of the tibial cutting jig.

Pearls

- The femoral pins are best placed in the metadiaphyseal junction, on the anteromedial border of the femur.
- The proximal tibial bone has a broad cancellous part, so the incidence of periprosthetic fractures is low.

Registration

- After fixing the arrays to the bones, the registration is performed as described by that particular navigation system.
- Registration of the femoral head, bony landmarks of the distal femur, proximal tibia, and ankle joint is done sequentially.
- Upon completion of the registration process, the navigation system reveals the overall coronal, axial, and sagittal plane deformity present.

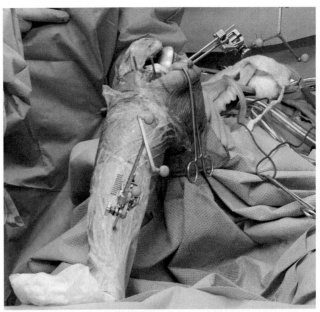

Fig. 2.12 An intraoperative picture depicting the arrays fixed in the distal femur within the surgical incision and in diaphyseal tibia, outside the surgical incision.

Steps of Registration

- Correct *placement* of camera unit in relation to arrays.
- Identify the *center of rotation of hip* joint for femoral head center.
- *Femoral landmarks registration:*
  - Femoral mechanical axis point.
  - Medial epicondylar point.
  - Lateral epicondylar point.
  - Anterior cortex point.
  - Whiteside line.
- *Femoral surface registration:*
  - Medial condyle.
  - Lateral condyle.
  - Anterior femoral cortex.
- *Verification* of the femoral model.
- *Tibial Malleoli registration:*
  - Medial malleolar point.
  - Lateral malleolar point.
- *Tibial landmark registration:*
  - Tibial mechanical axis point.
  - Medial tibial contour point.
  - Lateral tibial contour point.
  - Anterior tibial contour point.
  - Tibial AP direction.
- *Tibial surface registration:*
  - Medial tibial plateau.
  - Lateral tibial plateau.
  - Anterior tibial cortex.
- *Verification of the tibial model.*
- *Intraoperative kinematic graph.*

Correct Placement of the Camera Unit in Relation to the Arrays

- It is important to verify the placement and visualization of the arrays and camera unit in extension, flexion, internal rotation, and external rotation of the limb (**Fig. 2.13**).
- The arrays should be seen by the camera in all positions so that they remain visible even after correction of deformity.
- Both the arrays are spaced adequately and should not overlap each other (**Fig. 2.14**).

Identification of the Center of Rotation of the Hip Joint

- The foremost step in landmark registration is to accurately identify the center of rotation of the hip joint.
- The knee is flexed to 90 degrees, the hip is abducted, and a slow circular or elliptical rotational movement is executed (**Fig. 2.15**).
- The resultant motion is a conical one whose apex corresponds with the hip joint.

Pearls

The pelvis should be stabilized during this step.

- If the registration is incomplete or an unwanted movement of the pelvis occurs, then an error will be shown necessitating repetition of the process (**Fig. 2.16**).

Femoral Landmarks Registration

Femoral Mechanical Axis Point

- The first anatomical registration point is the femoral mechanical axis point, which is placed 1 cm above the femoral anterior cruciate ligament (ACL) insertion along the midline (**Fig. 2.17**).
- The pointer should be placed slightly medially, at the posterior aspect of the femoral notch point. It corresponds to the entry point in the conventional method.

Medial Epicondylar Point

- The medial epicondyle is felt as a rounded protrusion, on the medial side of the distal femur (**Fig. 2.18**).
- The groove is felt in the center, on which the landmark is registered.
- Care is to be exerted while performing the registration, as the epicondyle is relatively less prominent and covered with soft tissue.

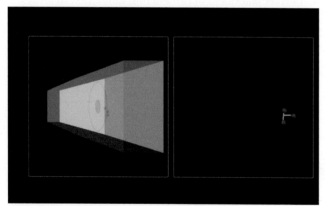

Fig. 2.13 After fixation of the arrays to the Schanz screws, the camera unit is so arranged that the arrays are in direct visual field of the camera.

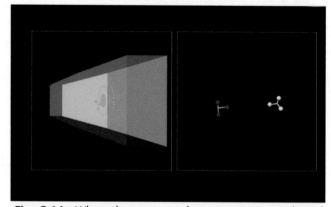

Fig. 2.14 When the arrays and camera unit are aligned correctly, the corresponding reference image occupies the central part of the screen.

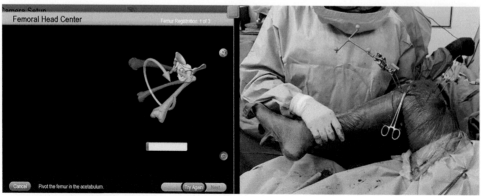

Fig. 2.15 Images depicting circumduction of the thigh to determine the center of rotation of the hip joint.

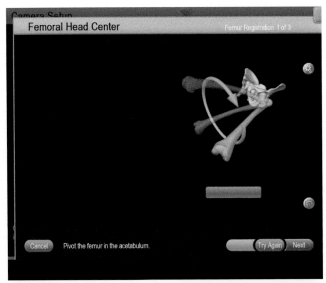

Fig. 2.16 The registration process ends with the completion of green bar.

- The medial and lateral epicondyles give the mediolateral dimension of the distal femur as well as determine the epicondylar axis, which assists navigation in interpreting the femoral component rotational alignment.[3]

Pitfalls

- In severely deformed or posttraumatic knees, it may be challenging to accurately identify and mark both the epicondyles.[4]
- This error may result in misinterpreted transepicondylar axis; hence, the surgeon should be cautious while using it as the main rotation reference point.

Lateral Epicondylar Point

- Anatomically, it is more prominent and present slightly lower on the mediolateral axis in comparison to the medial epicondyle (**Fig. 2.19**).
- It provides attachment to the fibular collateral ligament (FCL).

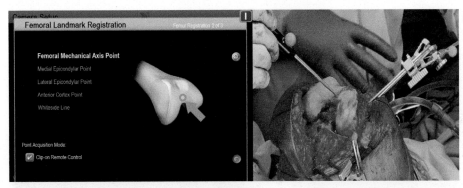

Fig. 2.17 Femoral mechanical axis point.

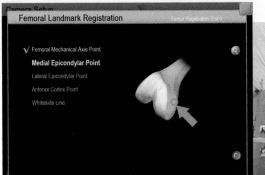

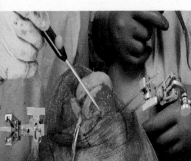

Fig. 2.18 The medial epicondylar point is marked, which is the attachment for the superficial part or "tendinous insertion" of the adductor magnus.

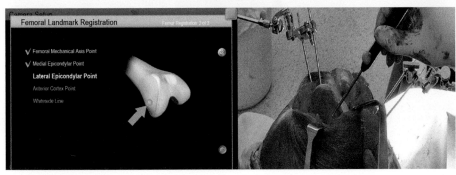

Fig. 2.19 The lateral epicondyle is present on the lateral side of the distal femur.

Anterior Cortex Point

- The anterior cortex is marked to determine the anterior extension of the distal femur (**Fig. 2.20**).
- It is the highest point on the lateral edge of the femur.
- It corresponds to the notch point on the anterior femoral cortex.

Whiteside Line

- The Whiteside line is also known as the anteroposterior (AP) axis of the knee (**Fig. 2.21**).
- It is marked as the deepest part in the intercondylar groove, above the intercondylar notch.
- This axis, along with the epicondylar axis, serves as the basis for deciding the femoral component rotation.
- The stylus needs to be held still while registering.

Femoral Surface Registration

Medial Condyle

- At first, a point is marked and then the stylus is moved over the entire medial condyle surface, ensuring that the whole condyle including the posterior surface is adequately "painted" (**Fig. 2.22**).
- The stylus is held like a pen and run over the entire medial condyle.
- The surgeon should avoid taking air points during the registration process, as it may depict false thickness of the femoral condyle (**Fig. 2.23**).
- The stylus is moved in a continuous motion without lifting it away from the bone.

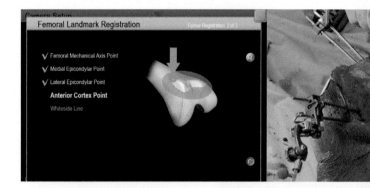

Fig. 2.20 Anterior cortex point.

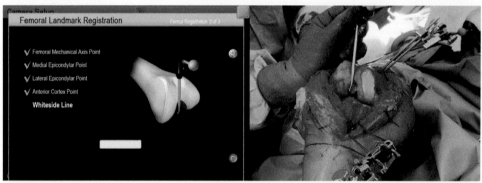

Fig. 2.21 Whiteside line.

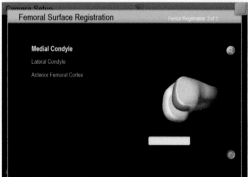
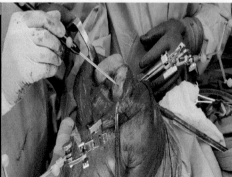

Fig. 2.22 Medial condyle femur.

- In the presence of severe cartilage loss or a patchy loss of cartilage, the stylus should include points on all the surfaces, as it helps in guiding the software to determine the required thickness of the bony cut.

Lateral Condyle

- The articular surface of the lateral femoral condyle is marked similarly (**Fig. 2.24**).
- The stylus should not overlap with the femoral array while registering.

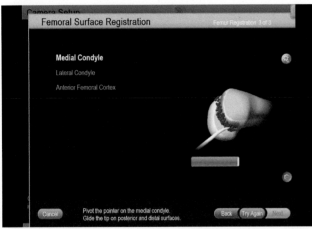

Fig. 2.23 Medial femoral condyle surface marking.

Anterior Femoral Cortex

- The last landmark during femoral registration is to paint the anterior femoral cortex (**Fig. 2.25**).

Verification of the Femoral Model

- The data entered into the navigation system is analyzed by the software and a resultant 3D image is created.
- The final step in the femoral registration is confirmation of registration and to verify its accuracy (**Fig. 2.26**).
- During this step, the pointer needs to be kept at any bony point over the femoral condylar or anterior cortical surface and pivoted in its place to acquire an accuracy checkpoint.
- Then the distance to the model is checked to ensure the accuracy of the femoral 3D model.

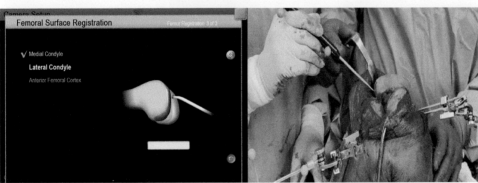

Fig. 2.24 Lateral condyle femur.

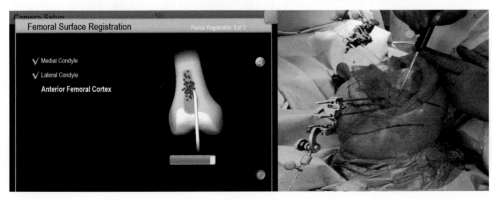

Fig. 2.25 Anterior femoral cortex surface marking.

Tibial Malleoli Registration

Medial Malleolar Point

- The first step in tibial registration is to mark the medial malleoli (**Fig. 2.27**).
- Registration is easier in lean patients.

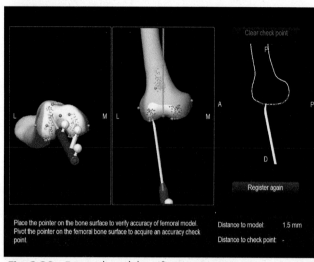

Fig. 2.26 Femoral model verification.

- In patients with morbid obesity or in those with ankle edema/deformity, accurate identification of the medial malleoli can be difficult.

Lateral Malleolar Point

- Subsequently, the lateral malleoli is marked, which is more prominent and easily palpable in comparison to the medial malleoli (**Fig. 2.28**).
- Both of these malleoli are the only bony landmarks that need to be marked above the skin.
- The remaining landmarks are identified and confirmed under direct vision, reducing the chances of inaccuracy.
- These bony landmarks decide the mechanical axis of the tibia, which forms the basis of the tibial cut.

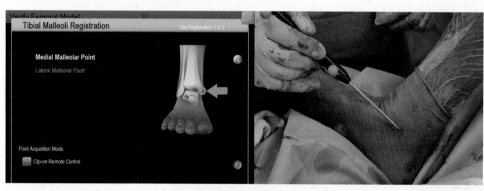

Fig. 2.27 Medial malleoli registration.

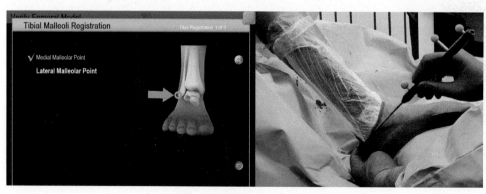

Fig. 2.28 Lateral malleoli registration.

Tibial Landmark Registration

Tibial Mechanical Axis Point

- The tibial mechanical axis point is marked at the *ACL footprint*, which is present just medial to the tibial spine (**Fig. 2.29**).

Medial Tibial Contour Point

- The medial tibial contour point is the medial-most extension of the tibial condyle (**Fig. 2.30**).

Lateral Tibial Contour Point

- The lateral tibial contour point is the lateral-most extension of the tibial condyle (**Fig. 2.31**).

- Keeping a right angle Hohmann retractor in the pocket between lateral condyle and patella may facilitate its registration.

Anterior Tibial Contour Point

- The anterior tibial contour point is the anterior extension of the tibial condylar surface (**Fig. 2.32**).

Tibial AP Direction

- The tibial AP direction refers to the axis made by joining the tibial attachments of posterior cruciate ligament (PCL), ACL, and the tibial tuberosity (**Fig. 2.33**).
- The stylus is kept horizontal so that all these three points lie in a straight line.

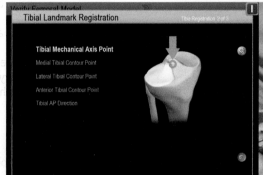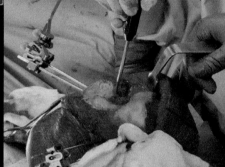

Fig. 2.29 Tibial mechanical axis.

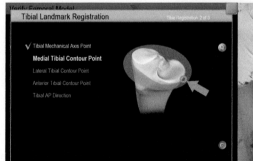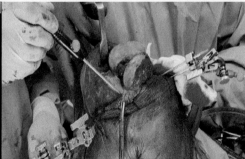

Fig. 2.30 Medial tibial contour point.

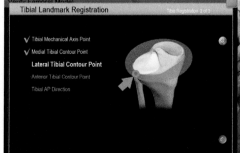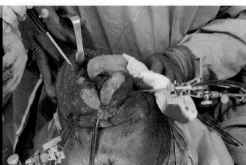

Fig. 2.31 Lateral tibial contour point.

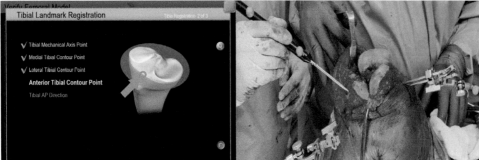

Fig. 2.32 Anterior tibial contour point.

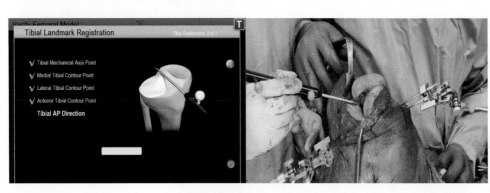

Fig. 2.33 Tibial anteroposterior (AP) direction.

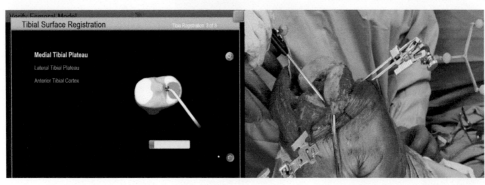

Fig. 2.34 Medial tibial condylar surface registration.

- This helps the computer software to determine the natural slope of tibia.

Tibial Surface Registration

Medial Tibial Plateau

- Similar to the femoral condylar surface, the medial tibial condylar surface is also registered (**Fig. 2.34**).
- The varus deformity is mainly on the tibial side, so in severe varus cases, the medial tibial condyle is worn off and has bone defect.

- Hence meticulous registration of the tibial surface, especially the deepest part of the condyle, is required.

Lateral Tibial Plateau

- The lateral tibial condyle is registered as the subsequent surgical step (**Fig. 2.35**).
- Care needs to be exerted in registering the lowest and the highest bony points on the lateral tibial plateau as the tibial cut height is measured from the highest point on the lateral tibial plateau.

Anterior Tibial Cortex

- The last landmark in tibial registration is the anterior tibial cortex registration (**Fig. 2.36**).
- Both the medial and lateral extensions of the anterior cortex are marked.

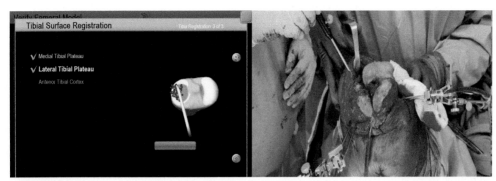

Fig. 2.35 Lateral tibial condyle registration.

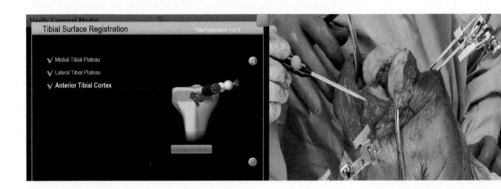

Fig. 2.36 Anterior tibial cortex registration.

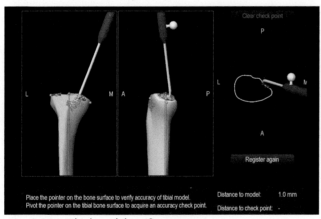

Fig. 2.37 Tibial model verification.

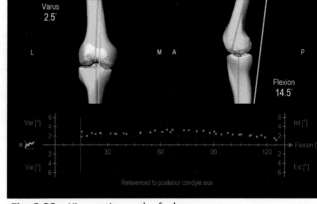

Fig. 2.38 Kinematic graph of a knee.

- Care has to be taken in marking the lateral extension, as it lies below the patellar tendon.
- This landmark helps determine the thickness of the tibial cut.

Verification of the Tibial Model

- Similar to the femoral registration, the navigation software interprets the data fed and forms a 3D image (**Fig. 2.37**).
- The surgeon needs to verify the accuracy by keeping the stylus over any two bony points and registering them by pivoting the stylus to obtain an accuracy checkpoint.

Intraoperative Kinematics Graph

- This kinematic graph reveals the deformity in coronal and sagittal planes and the behavior of coronal plane deformity throughout the range of motion (**Fig. 2.38**).
- The purple dots in the image represent the preoperative position of the knee joint during the entire range of movement.
- The horizontal axis determines the range of movement from 0 to 120 degrees and beyond.
- The vertical axis on the left in this graph represents the coronal alignment of the knee.
- Every knee has a unique pattern of coronal plane deformity as it moves from an extended position to complete flexion.[5]

- Such patterns are impossible to identify with naked eyes.
- Computer navigation or robotics helps in identification of these unique patterns.
- It is important to check the coronal plane deformity in complete extension, at 30, 60, 90, and 120 degrees of flexion.
- The medial soft tissues in a varus knee and the lateral soft tissues in a valgus knee should be judiciously released to balance the knee. Overzealous release often causes flexion instability.[6]
- Navigation helps in individualizing the soft tissue releases required for each knee to balance the mediolateral gaps in extension and flexion.
- Broadly, knees can have following kinematic patterns[7] (**Table 2.2**).

Type 1

- Deformity increases or remains the same throughout ROM (**Fig. 2.39**).
- Interpretation:
  - This graph shows that knee remains in varus as knee flexes.
  - Medial gap will remain tight with flexion in comparison to lateral gap and mediolateral gap difference would be more than 2 mm.

- Method to correct:
  - Requires soft tissue release for coronal correction in extension and flexion.
  - Medial and posteromedial soft tissue releases with tibia reduction osteotomy may be required to balance the gap.
  - Femoral external rotation can be increased by 1 to 2 degrees to compensate for tight medial gap in flexion.
  - In valgus deformity, increasingly tight lateral gap in flexion may need popliteus release.

Pearls

Authors prefer popliteus pie crusting with 16-gauge needle instead of complete release.

Type 2

- Deformity decreases but does not reach neutral on knee flexion (**Fig. 2.40**).
- Interpretation:
  - As knee flexes, varus decreases but doesn't correct fully.
  - Medial gap will remain tighter in flexion as compared to lateral gap but mediolateral gap difference would be less than 2 mm.

Table 2.2 Knee classification on the basis of kinematic pattern

Main group	Coronal deformity as the knee flexes from extension to 90-degree flexion and beyond
Varus/Valgus	
1	Deformity increases or remains the same throughout the range of motion (ROM)
2	Deformity decreases but does not reach neutral
3	Deformity decreases and reaches neutral
4	Deformity becomes opposite deformity (varus becomes valgus and valgus becomes varus)

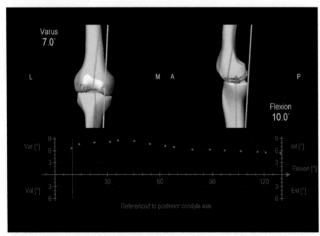

Fig. 2.39 Type 1 kinematic graph.

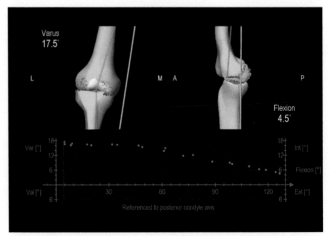

Fig. 2.40 Type 2 kinematic graph.

- Method to correct:
  - Most common pattern encountered.
  - Requires soft tissue releases to balance coronal deformity in both extension and flexion though (extension>flexion).
- Femoral external rotation can be increased to balance the mediolateral gap in flexion, thus limiting the amount of soft tissue releases required to balance mediolateral gap in flexion.

Type 3

- Deformity decreases and reaches neutral on deep flexion (**Fig. 2.41**).
- Interpretation:
  - Coronal deformity is more in extension in comparison to flexion and becomes neutral at terminal ROM.
  - When knee is extended, there is tight medial gap in comparison to lateral gap.
  - As the knee flexes, coronal deformity becomes neutral or mediolateral gap equalizes.
- Method to correct:
  - Requires only posteromedial soft tissue releases for tight gap in extension.
  - Keep external femoral rotation to 3 degrees to transepicondylar axis.
  - Overzealous anteromedial release can lead to opening up of medial gap in flexion.

Type 4

- Deformity becomes opposite deformity (varus becomes valgus and valgus becomes varus) (**Fig. 2.42**).
- Interpretation:
  - In this pattern of deformity, knee changes behavior in flexion which is difficult to interpret by conventional method.
  - Coronal plane deformity changes from varus to valgus or valgus to varus as the knee flexes.

- So if there is tight medial gap in extension, medial gap opens up in flexion.
- Method to correct:
  - Requires none or minimal soft tissue release, especially of anteromedial structures, as it can lead to opening of medial space and asymmetric flexion instability.
  - Overrelease can lead to flexion instability.
  - Keep femoral external rotation at 3 degrees.

Navigation Cutting Blocks

- The conventional cutting guides are positioned with the help of computer navigation, to obtain the desired bony cuts.
- Navigation enables the surgeon to check the alignment in all three planes (coronal, sagittal, and axial).
- The femoral and tibia cuts can be titrated in terms of the thickness and its orientation in all the planes.

Distal Femoral Planning

- The subsequent step is to plan a resection level of the distal femur, which is decided according to the deformity and thickness of the distal femur prosthesis (**Fig. 2.43**).
- Usually, 9.5 mm of distal femur cut is taken, in 1 to 3 degrees of flexion.
- Distal femur cut is the most important cut as it selectively influences the extension gap only as compared to tibial cut which influences both the gaps equally. Hence, it is extremely important to calculate the correct resection depth of the distal femur as more resection can lead to recurvatum deformity and elevation of the joint line.
- Distal femur can show 2 variations with respect to cartilage loss.
  - Lateral femoral condyle with intact cartilage is thicker than the worn medial side and 9.5 mm is calculated from the lateral side.

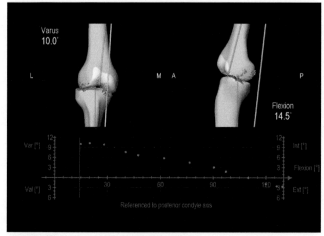

Fig. 2.41 Type 3 kinematic graph.

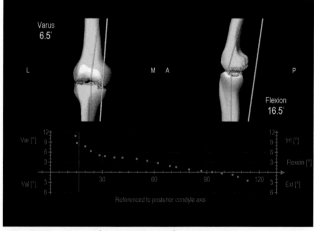

Fig. 2.42 Type 4 kinematic graph.

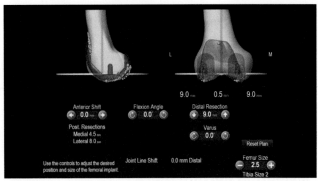

Fig. 2.43 Distal femur planning.

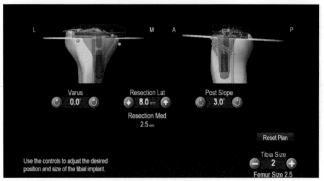

Fig. 2.44 Tibial implant planning.

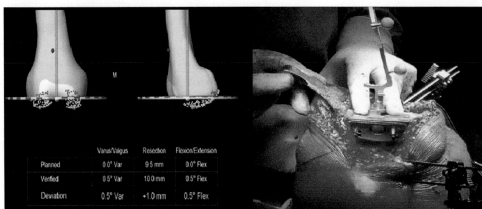

Fig. 2.45 Distal femur resection verification.

- Lateral and medial side may be equal despite cartilage loss on medial side. Here, 7 mm is resected on medial side to account for 2- to 3 mm of cartilage loss.

Tibial planning

- Similar to the distal femur, the proximal tibial cut is also planned in all three planes (**Fig. 2.44**).

Pearls

The authors recommend that the tibial bone cut should always be checked manually with an angel wing or measuring stylus before executing it.

Verification of Cuts

- Through navigation, the bony cuts can be verified in all the three planes.
- The verification steps reveal the potential deviations from the desired positioning through real-time feedback, making it easy to evaluate if the deviation can be accepted or needs a reassessment of the cut.

Verification of Distal Femoral Resection

- The femoral array is placed along with a cut array on the femoral cut surface (**Fig. 2.45**).

Verification of Tibial Resection

- The tibial array is placed along with a cut array on the tibial cut surface (**Fig. 2.46**).

Principles

- Achieving the correct tibial slope is an essential requirement to maintain the flexion gap, especially in cruciate-retaining (CR) knees.
- Computer navigation accurately predicts and provides the surgeon with an indispensable tool to titrate the posterior slope, along with achieving a neutral tibial cut in the coronal plane.[8]

Gap Balancing

- After completion of all the bony cuts, navigation reveals the medial and lateral gaps accurately with trial prosthetic components (**Fig. 2.47** and **Fig. 2.48**).[9]

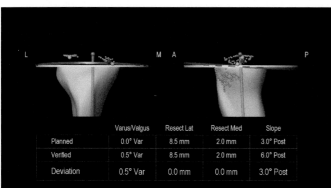

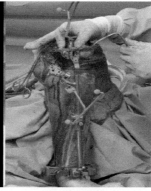

	Varus/Valgus	Resect Lat	Resect Med	Slope
Planned	0.0° Var	8.5 mm	2.0 mm	3.0° Post
Verified	0.5° Var	8.5 mm	2.0 mm	6.0° Post
Deviation	0.5° Var	0.0 mm	0.0 mm	3.0° Post

Fig. 2.46 Tibial resection verification.

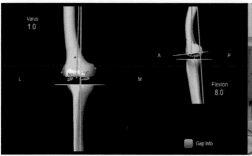

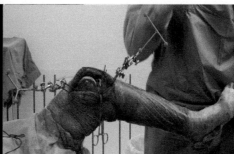

Fig. 2.47 Alignment with trial components in situ.

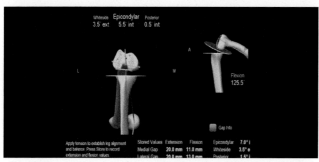

Fig. 2.48 Navigation demonstrating the alignment, medial, and lateral gap values in flexion and extension.

Principles

- Navigation quantifies these gaps throughout the range of motion of the knee, whereas in conventional method the surgeon can only check the gaps in full extension and 90-degree flexion. Thus, computer navigation aids in the better titration of soft tissue release.
- Navigation also helps in prediction of the final range of movement of the knee.

Final Alignment

- Navigation helps determine the overall alignment with trial prosthetic components.
- Hence the need for final fine tuning of soft tissue balance can be done under navigation guidance.
- The surgeon can also verify and document the final limb alignment after the implantation of the prosthesis.

Points to Remember

- Every knee has unique kinematic behavior as it moves from extension to flexion.
- Varus knees may show increase or decrease in varus as they go in flexion. This determines the soft tissue releases required. For varus knees which remain in varus with knee flexion, reduction osteotomy along with posteromedial soft tissue releases will be required to correct the deformity.
- Rotation can also be increased by 2 degrees to facilitate harmonious soft tissue balance.
- Conversely, for knees in which varus corrects fully in flexion, no anterior release should be performed lest it leads to flexion instability. Only posteromedial structures should be released to correct varus deformity in extension.
- Similarly, valgus deformity may increase or decrease in flexion.
- If valgus deformity increases in flexion, popliteus release may be required to correct valgus deformity in flexion.
- Mostly valgus deformity corrects itself in flexion; hence, only ilio tibial band and posterolateral capsule may need release to correct the deformity in extension.
- Some element of deformity may persist after trial reduction which may need additional fine-tuning of balance like pie crusting of medial collateral ligament in varus knees.
- Final objective is to correct the deformity within 3 degrees of coronal plane in extension and obtain harmonious balance in flexion within 2 mm difference in mediolateral gaps.

References

1. Bae DK, Song SJ. Computer assisted navigation in knee arthroplasty. Clin Orthop Surg 2011;3(4):259–267

2. Pitto RP, Graydon AJ, Bradley L, Malak SF, Walker CG, Anderson IA. Accuracy of a computer-assisted navigation system for total knee replacement. J Bone Joint Surg Br 2006;88(5):601–605

3. Stiehl JB, Abbott BD. Morphology of the transepicondylar axis and its application in primary and revision total knee arthroplasty. J Arthroplasty 1995;10(6):785–789

4. Castelli CC, Falvo DA, Iapicca ML, Gotti V. Rotational alignment of the femoral component in total knee arthroplasty. Ann Transl Med 2016;4(1):4

5. Siston RA, Giori NJ, Goodman SB, Delp SL. Intraoperative passive kinematics of osteoarthritic knees before and after total knee arthroplasty. J Orthop Res 2006;24(8):1607–1614

6. Ghosh KM, Blain AP, Longstaff L, Rushton S, Amis AA, Deehan DJ. Can we define envelope of laxity during navigated knee arthroplasty? Knee Surg Sports Traumatol Arthrosc 2014;22(8):1736–1743

7. Deep K, Picard F, Baines J. Dynamic knee behaviour: does the knee deformity change as it is flexed-an assessment and classification with computer navigation. Knee Surg Sports Traumatol Arthrosc 2016;24(11):3575–3583

8. Di Benedetto P, Di Benedetto ED, Buttironi MM, et al. Computer assisted total knee arthroplasty: a real navigation to better results? Acta Biomed 2017;88(2S):48–53

9. Lee DH, Park JH, Song DI, Padhy D, Jeong WK, Han SB. Accuracy of soft tissue balancing in TKA: comparison between navigation-assisted gap balancing and conventional measured resection. Knee Surg Sports Traumatol Arthrosc 2010;18(3):381–387

Computer-Navigated TKR for Varus and Associated Sagittal Deformity

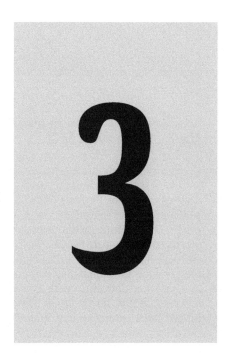

Anoop Jhurani and Piyush Agarwal

Introduction

- Varus is the commonest manifestation of the arthritic process resulting from the weight-bearing axis passing through the medial compartment of the knee joint.[1,2]
- Varus is mostly described as a standalone deformity but our data suggests that it seldom presents as a uniplanar deformity.
- In about 85% of cases, varus is associated with some FFD and in 15% cases with hyperextension deformity.
- This chapter not only deals with correction of varus deformity but also its association, interplay and correction of sagittal plane deformity (fixed flexion deformity [FFD]/hyperextension).
- As the varus deformity progresses, it achieves a biplanar dimension, manifesting as a varus-flexion or varus-recurvatum deformity.[3,4]
- Computer navigation assists in the correct estimation of the varus deformity in the coronal plane and the associated flexion/recurvatum deformity in the sagittal plane.[5]
- Navigation also demonstrates the overall fixed and dynamic deformity throughout the range of motion (ROM) of the knee.
- In the majority of the cases, varus deformity gradually corrects itself as the knee flexes, thus requiring less soft tissue release of anteromedial structures to obtain ligament balance.[6]
- However, in patients with resistant varus deformity, a greater extent of soft tissue release or a reduction osteotomy may be required to achieve optimal alignment and balance.[7]

- Based on the severity of varus, the sequence of soft tissue release followed by the authors is[8]:
  - Subperiosteal elevation of deep medial collateral ligament (MCL).
  - Posteromedial (PM) capsule.
  - Semimembranosus.
  - Reductional osteotomy of tibia.
  - Pie crusting of superficial MCL.
  - Sliding medial epicondylar osteotomy.
- Based on its association of sagittal component, varus deformity can be divided as:
  - Varus with FFD.
    - Varus ≈ FFD.
    - Varus < FFD.
    - Varus > FFD.
  - Varus with a recurvatum deformity:
    - Varus ≈ Recurvatum.
    - Varus < Recurvatum.
    - Varus > Recurvatum.

Principle for Biplanar Deformity Correction

- The authors have observed that in the knees with a biplanar deformity, the correction of a coronal plane deformity also results in the correction of the concomitant sagittal plane deformity in equal measure. Thus a 10-degree varus correction will also correct about 10 degree of associated flexion deformity.

- The release of tight PM structures relaxes the posterior capsule, leading to an increase in the extension gap.
- The surgeon should be aware of this possible gain in the extension gap while planning the distal femur resection.

Algorithm for Planning Distal Femur Cut in Varus Knee with FFD

- A varus-flexion deformity is caused by the contracture of the PM structures and the joint capsule, leading to the progression of the flexion deformity as the arthritic process increases in severity.
- In a biplanar deformity with equal angulation in both the planes (flexion ≈ varus), PM soft tissue release for varus correction corrects the flexion deformity, thus obviating the need for additional distal femur cut (**Table 3.1**).
- In a biplanar deformity with flexion > varus, the distal femur resection needs to be increased to compensate for the tight extension gap. This should not be done in the presence of large osteophytes in the posterior recess, as their removal also increases the extension space and corrects flexion deformity.
- In knees with varus > flexion deformity, the distal femur resection needs to be decreased by 1 to 2 mm to compensate for the potential overcorrection in the sagittal plane following the releases for varus correction.

Table 3.1 Distal femur cut in biplanar deformity

Varus (degrees)	FFD (degrees)	Distal femur cut (for S&N)
10	10	9.5 mm (regular)
20	10	8.5–9 mm (less)
10	20	10.5–11 mm (more)

Abbreviation: FFD, fixed flexion deformity.

Pearls

Such seemingly minor adjustments in the distal femur cut are quite significant to achieve the correct sagittal plane alignment and to balance the knee in both planes.

Varus with Fixed Flexion Deformity

- Varus ≈ FFD.
- Varus > FFD.
- Varus < FFD.

Varus ≈ FFD (10 degrees)

- The full-length radiographs of the lower limb with anteroposterior (AP) and lateral views of the left knee joint (**Fig. 3.1**).
- X-rays shows tricompartmental osteoarthritis with mild varus deformity.
- The kinematic analysis of this patient demonstrates a varus deformity of 10 degrees with 9.5 degrees of flexion in the sagittal plane (**Fig. 3.2**).
- The kinematic graph shows uncorrectable varus during the entire arc of movement. (Purple dotted line in **Fig. 3.2**.)
- This suggests that the medial gap is consistently tight which may need PM soft tissue release and downsizing of the tibial tray.
- The intraoperative navigation values show normal distal femur cut (**Fig. 3.3**).
- In such cases, the femoral component can be externally rotated to 5 to 6 degrees with respect to posterior condylar axis to balance the tight medial gap in flexion (**Fig. 3.4**).

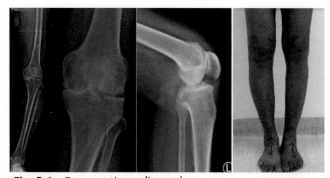

Fig. 3.1 Preoperative radiographs.

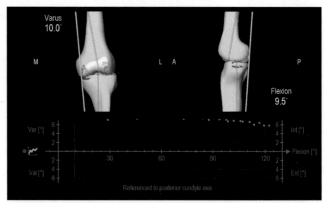

Fig. 3.2 Initial limb alignment and kinematics.

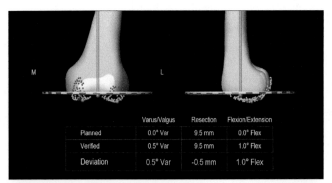

Fig. 3.3 Distal femur cut verification.

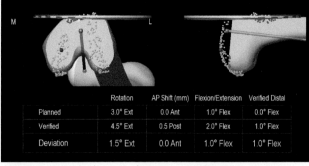

Fig. 3.4 Femoral external rotation verification.

- The femoral component rotation should be individualized in each case.
- Aligning the component in 3-degree external rotation as a routine in all the cases might lead to a tight medial gap and loose lateral gap, requiring unnecessary soft tissue releases and tibial downsizing for balancing the knee (**Fig. 3.5**).
- The femoral component rotation depends upon the following factors:
  - Knee kinematics.
  - Lateral joint space opening.
  - Bone loss due to arthritis.
  - Femoral component size.
  - Ligamentous laxity.

- The navigation values show the verification of the proximal tibial cut (**Fig. 3.6**).
- In a varus deformity, the medial tibial condyle gets worn off. Hence the lateral tibial resection is more than that of the medial tibial condyle.
- Navigation predicts the ideal thickness of the tibial bony cut by considering the posterior slope required to balance the knee.

- Occasionally, navigation doesn't predict the true thickness of the proximal tibial cut as required.
- The authors recommend manual verification of the thickness of the tibial resection both before and after executing the tibial cut.

- Verification of the thickness of the tibial bone resected with a Vernier caliper (**Fig. 3.7**).

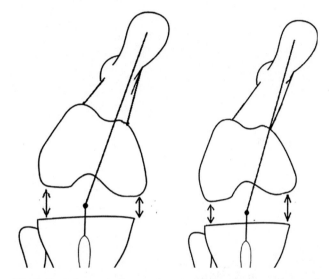

Fig. 3.5 Schematic figures demonstrating the importance of femoral component rotation in determining the mediolateral flexion gap.

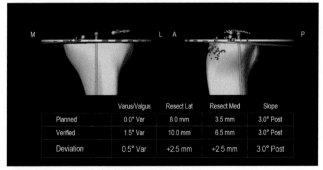

Fig. 3.6 Proximal tibia cut verification.

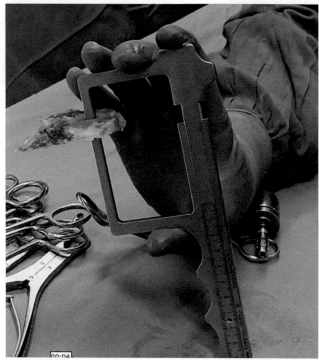

Fig. 3.7 Proximal tibia cut.

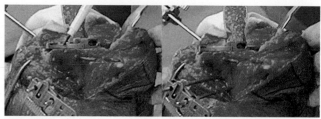

Fig. 3.8 Tibial baseplate kept in external rotation with reference to tibial tuberosity.

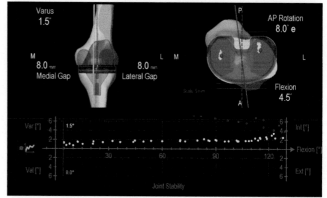

Fig. 3.9 Final limb alignment and kinematics.

- The PM soft tissue release required for the residual varus correction.
- Clinical pictures depicting the tibial tray kept in external rotation (**Fig. 3.8**).
- The AP axis of the tibial tray should be in line with the tibial tuberosity.
- The postoperative navigation graph showing the correction of deformity in both the sagittal and coronal planes (**Fig. 3.9**).
- There was a residual flexion of 4.5 degrees, with a gap difference of <2 mm throughout the ROM of the knee.
- The postoperative AP and lateral X-ray views of the knee joint showing well-placed femoral and tibial prosthesis components with corrected limb alignment (**Fig. 3.10**).

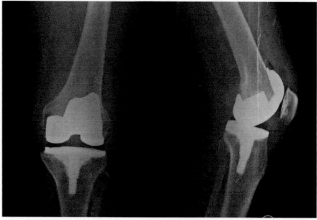

Fig. 3.10 Postoperative radiographs.

Varus ≈ FFD (20 degrees)

- The preoperative radiographs and clinical images reveal a severe varus and flexion deformity with laterally subluxed tibia (**Fig. 3.11** and **Fig. 3.12**).
- The patient had a history of bipolar hemiarthroplasty 8 years back, which further emphasizes the need for using navigation to perform total knee replacement (TKR).
- The preoperative kinematic analysis suggesting a severe varus and flexion deformity (**Fig. 3.13**).
- The extent of varus deformity was nearly as much as the flexion deformity.
- Laterally subluxed tibia can be appreciated in 3D reconstructed image.
- As varus equals FFD, normal resection of the distal femur was required to balance the extension gap with the flexion gap (**Fig. 3.14**).
- It is important to maintain the standard external rotation of the femoral prosthesis, as the loss of the cartilage over the posterior medial femoral condyle in severe varus knees may lead to increased external rotation (**Fig. 3.15**).
- The Whiteside line along with TEA is used to reconfirm femoral component rotation (**Fig. 3.16**).
- Under-resection of the proximal tibia was performed to balance the flexion and extension gaps with a 9-mm insert (**Fig. 3.17** and **Fig. 3.18**).
- Authors advise that the flexion and extension gaps should be reassessed after the PM soft tissue release, before proceeding with the proximal tibial cut (**Fig. 3.19**).
- The postoperative kinematic image showing complete correction of the biplanar deformity with balanced gaps throughout the knee ROM (**Fig. 3.20**).
- The postoperative radiograph demonstrates a well-aligned femoral and tibial component with corrected limb alignment (**Fig. 3.21**).
- A tibial stem was used to facilitate load shearing and to reduce stress on the tibial baseplate.

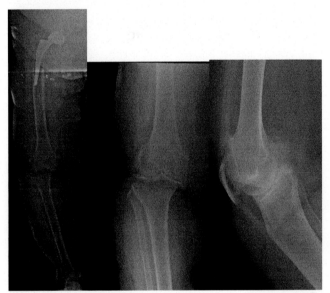

Fig. 3.11 Preoperative radiographs.

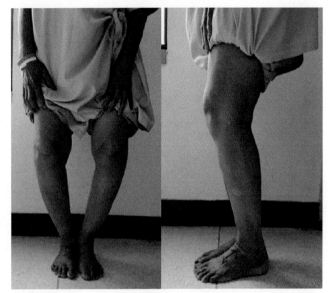

Fig. 3.12 Image of the patient.

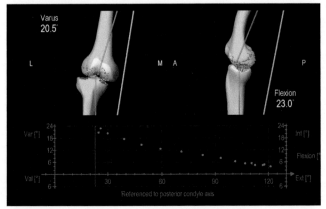

Fig. 3.13 Initial limb alignment and kinematics.

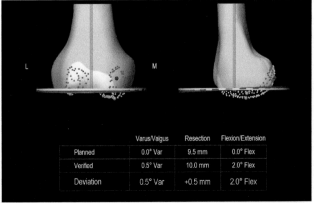

Fig. 3.14 Distal femur cut verification.

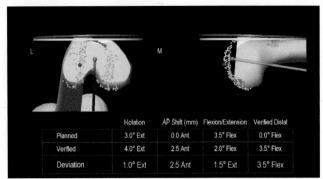

	Rotation	AP Shift (mm)	Flexion/Extension	Verified Distal
Planned	3.0° Ext	0.0 Ant	3.5° Flex	0.0° Flex
Verified	4.0° Ext	2.5 Ant	2.0° Flex	3.5° Flex
Deviation	1.0° Ext	2.5 Ant	1.5° Ext	3.5° Flex

Fig. 3.15   Femoral external rotation verification.

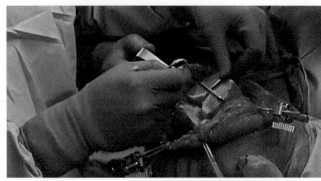

Fig. 3.16   Whiteside side marked over distal femur.

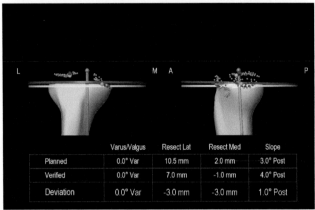

	Varus/Valgus	Resect Lat	Resect Med	Slope
Planned	0.0° Var	10.5 mm	2.0 mm	3.0° Post
Verified	0.0° Var	7.0 mm	-1.0 mm	4.0° Post
Deviation	0.0° Var	-3.0 mm	-3.0 mm	1.0° Post

Fig. 3.17   Proximal tibia cut verification.

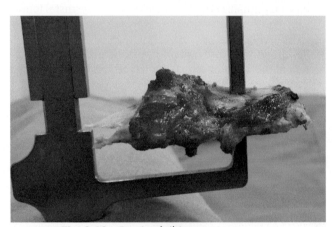

Fig. 3.18   Proximal tibia cut.

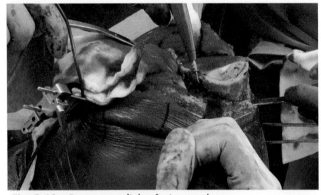

Fig. 3.19   Posteromedial soft tissue release.

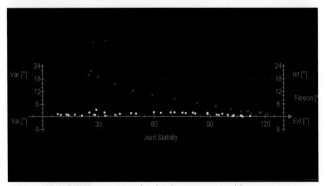

Fig. 3.20   Postoperative limb alignment and kinematics.

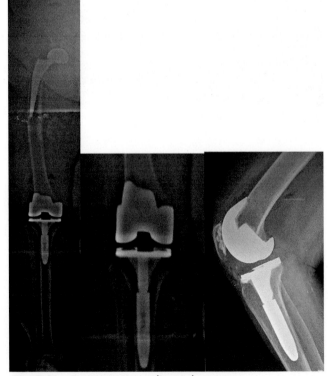

Fig. 3.21   Postoperative radiographs.

Varus < FFD

- The preoperative radiographs suggest a moderate varus deformity with the opening of the lateral joint space (**Fig. 3.22** and **Fig. 3.23**).
- The preoperative kinematics graph shows partial correction of the varus deformity with knee flexion (**Fig. 3.24**).
- FFD (20 degrees) is more than the varus deformity (13 degrees).
- An additional distal femur resection was performed to gain the extension gap (**Fig. 3.25**).
- If there are large osteophytes tightening the posterior capsule, then they should be removed first, extension gap should be reassessed before proceeding for extra distal femur cut.

- A measured proximal tibial resection with a normal posterior slope was planned to balance the flexion gap (**Fig. 3.26**).
  - A 20-gauge needle was used for MCL pie crusting in this patient (**Fig. 3.27**).
  - Authors reserve MCL pie crusting only for cases where the varus deformity is not correctable in flexion.
  - 10 to 12 needle pricks were given in anterior fibers of MCL to facilitate easy insertion of the insert.
  - This step should be guarded to prevent over release and instability.
- The postoperative kinematics demonstrate complete correction of the biplanar deformity (**Fig. 3.28**).
- The postoperative radiographs show well-aligned prosthetic components (**Fig. 3.29**).

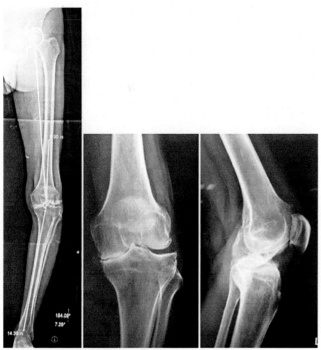

Fig. 3.22 Preoperative radiographs.

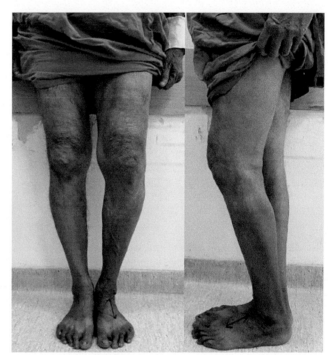

Fig. 3.23 Image of the patient.

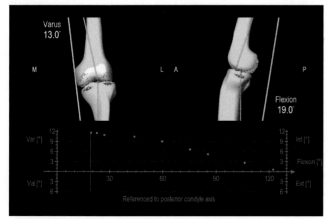

Fig. 3.24 Initial limb alignment and kinematics.

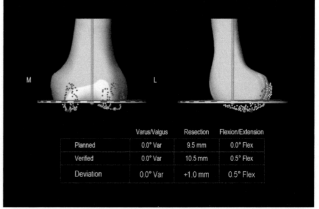

Fig. 3.25 Distal femur cut verification.

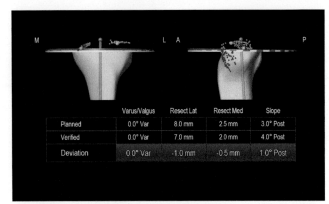

Fig. 3.26 Proximal tibia cut verification.

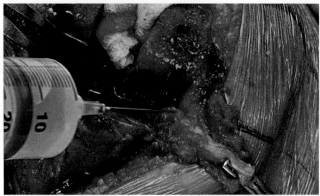

Fig. 3.27 Medial collateral ligament (MCL) pie crusting.

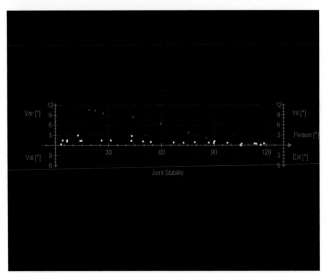

Fig. 3.28 Postoperative limb alignment and kinematics.

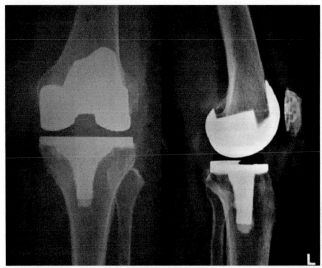

Fig. 3.29 Postoperative radiographs.

Varus > FFD

- The preoperative radiographs showing a moderate varus deformity with subluxed joint (**Fig. 3.30** and **Fig. 3.31**).
- The preoperative kinematic analysis showing 11.5-degree varus associated with almost neutral sagittal alignment (**Fig. 3.32**).
- Under resection of distal femur was performed considering varus correction will increase extension gap (**Fig. 3.33**).
- Measured tibial resection was done to create adequate gap for insert (**Fig. 3.34**).
- Kinematic analysis showing residual varus flexion deformity with tight medial gap (**Fig. 3.35**).
- At this stage, there is no need for additional distal femur resection as the correction of residual varus would correct the remaining FFD.
- Tight medial gap causing lateral opening and FFD (**Fig. 3.36**).

- Tibial baseplate is downsized and PM bone is marked (**Fig. 3.37**).
- Tibial baseplate should not be downsized so much so that it sinks in soft cancellous bone of lateral condyle.
- Tibial baseplate should sit on lateral tibial cortex and shouldn't overhang medially.
- PM bone resection with help of saw to relax the PM soft tissue structures (**Fig. 3.38**).

Pearls

Whenever a saw is used for reduction osteotomy, MCL should be carefully protected.

- Gap balanced with 1 to 2 mm lateral opening and smooth reduction in flexion (**Fig. 3.39**).
- Postoperative kinematic analysis showing complete correction of biplanar deformity without additional bone resection (**Fig. 3.40**).

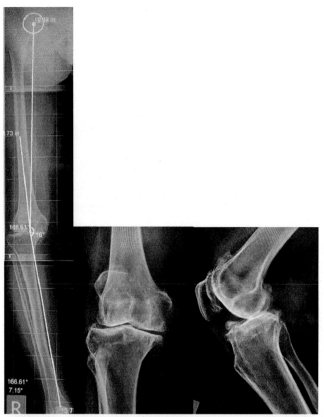

Fig. 3.30 Preoperative radiographs.

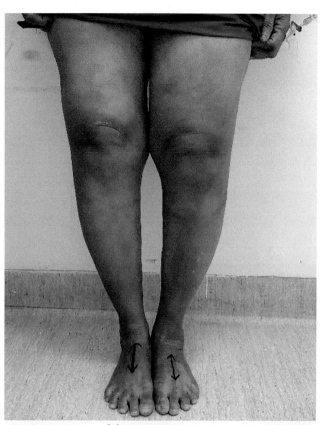

Fig. 3.31 Image of the patient.

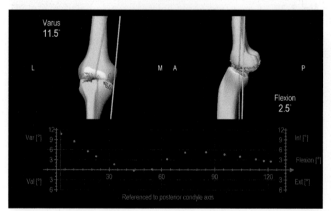

Fig. 3.32 Initial limb alignment and kinematics.

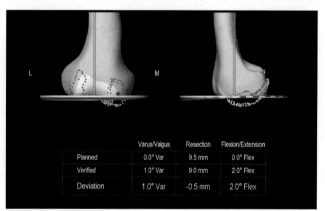

Fig. 3.33 Distal femur cut verification.

	Varus/Valgus	Resection	Flexion/Extension
Planned	0.0° Var	9.5 mm	0.0° Flex
Verified	1.0° Var	9.0 mm	2.0° Flex
Deviation	1.0° Var	-0.5 mm	2.0° Flex

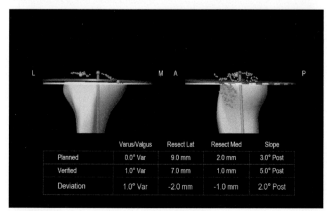

Fig. 3.34 Proximal tibia cut verification.

	Varus/Valgus	Resect Lat	Resect Med	Slope
Planned	0.0° Var	9.0 mm	2.0 mm	3.0° Post
Verified	1.0° Var	7.0 mm	1.0 mm	5.0° Post
Deviation	1.0° Var	-2.0 mm	-1.0 mm	2.0° Post

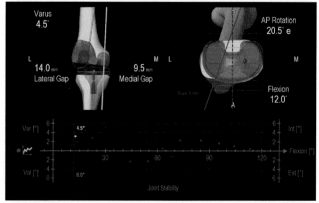

Fig. 3.35 Postoperative limb alignment and kinematics.

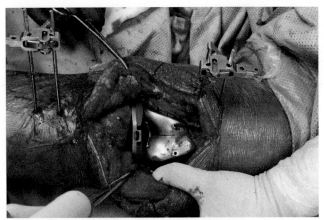

Fig. 3.36 Tight medial gap with lateral laxity.

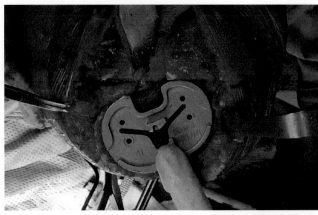

Fig. 3.37 Posteromedial reduction osteotomy of tibia.

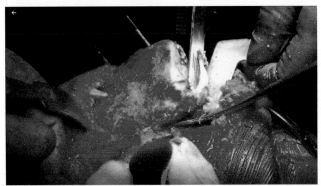

Fig. 3.38 Removal of posteromedial bone.

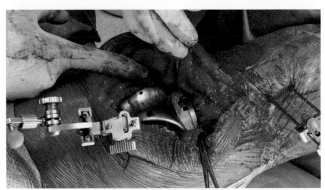

Fig. 3.39 Correction of mediolateral gap imbalance.

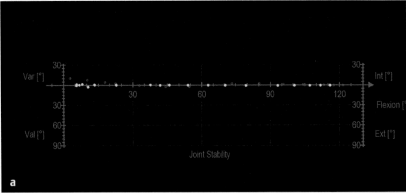
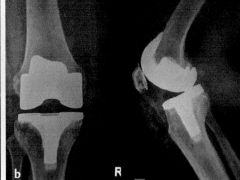

Fig. 3.40 **(a, b)** Postoperative kinematics and radiographs showing balanced knee with well-fixed component.

Varus >> FFD

- The preoperative radiographs and clinical images of the left knee demonstrate subluxed knee with profound varus deformity (**Fig. 3.41** and **Fig. 3.42**).
- A constrained prosthesis should be available as a backup for such cases.
- The preoperative kinematic analysis demonstrated a subluxed knee with more than 20-degree varus associated with minimal flexion deformity (**Fig. 3.43**).
- The navigation values depict conservative distal femur resection. This is because extension gap opens up after correction of varus deformity (**Fig. 3.44**).
- A conservative proximal tibial cut was planned to manage the gaps (**Fig. 3.45**).
- Intraoperatively, despite downsizing the tibial component and performing an extensive PM soft tissue release, there was lateral joint space opening with a tight medial gap (**Fig. 3.46**).

- The navigation screen demonstrated a residual 8.5-degree varus alignment despite performing the soft tissue releases (**Fig. 3.47**).
- A sliding medial epicondylar osteotomy was performed under navigation guidance to correct the residual varus deformity (**Fig. 3.48**).
- The medial epicondyle was fixed in a position where the knee was stable and mechanically aligned in the coronal and sagittal planes, with the help of computer navigation.[9]
- The navigation graph shows complete correction of varus deformity (**Fig. 3.49**).
- The postoperative radiographs show correction of varus deformity with well-fixed medial epicondylar osteotomy (**Fig. 3.50**).
- The authors prefer to utilize a tibial stem in such cases to provide extra stability and to distribute stress on weight-bearing.

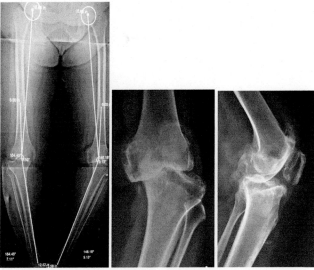

Fig. 3.41 Preoperative radiographs.

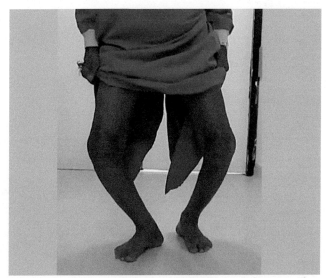

Fig. 3.42 Clinical image of the patient.

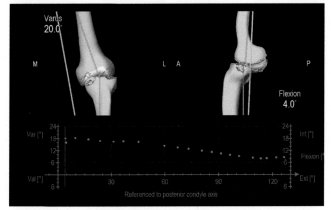

Fig. 3.43 Initial limb alignment and kinematics.

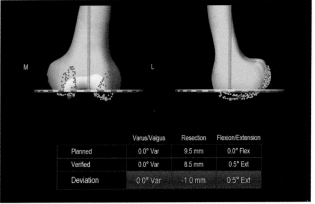

Fig. 3.44 Distal femur cut verification.

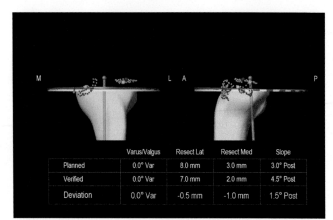

Fig. 3.45 Proximal tibia cut verification.

	Varus/Valgus	Resect Lat	Resect Med	Slope
Planned	0.0° Var	8.0 mm	3.0 mm	3.0° Post
Verified	0.0° Var	7.0 mm	2.0 mm	4.5° Post
Deviation	0.0° Var	-0.5 mm	-1.0 mm	1.5° Post

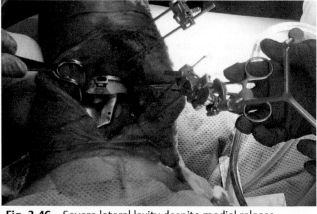

Fig. 3.46 Severe lateral laxity despite medial release.

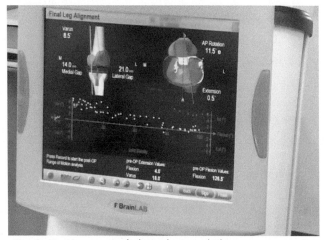

Fig. 3.47 Severe mediolateral gap imbalance on navigation screen.

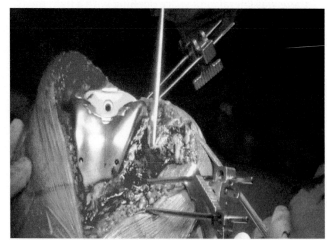

Fig. 3.48 Medial epicondyle osteotomy.

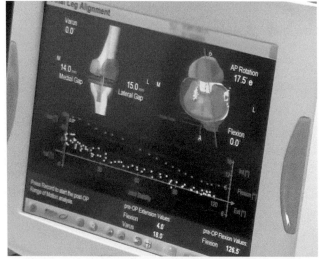

Fig. 3.49 Correction of mediolateral gaps and deformity.

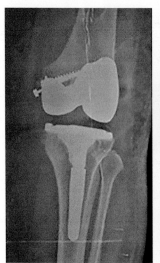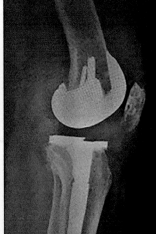

Fig. 3.50 Postoperative radiographs.

Varus with Hyperextension (Recurvatum) Deformity

- A varus deformity along with recurvatum can be subtle and occult finding. Careful gait examination is required to identify it preoperatively.
- Hyperextension associated with varus deformity can be due to cartilage loss or soft tissue laxity.
- Hyperextension is prone to recurrence and subsequent failure. Thus, it is important to identify it preoperatively.
- Authors recommend to keep these knees in 5 to 7 degrees of flexion to prevent recurrence of recurvatum.

Varus with Recurvatum Deformity

- Varus ≈ Recurvatum.
- Varus > Recurvatum.
- Varus < Recurvatum.

Algorithm for Planning Distal Femur Cut in Varus Knee with Hyperextension

- When varus is associated with recurvatum, distal femur and tibial cut need to be conservative.
- If recurvatum > varus deformity, the distal femur resection needs to be decreased by a 1 to 2 mm to tighten the extension gap. The authors' aim to achieve a 5 to 7 degrees of flexion postoperatively in patients presenting with a recurvatum deformity as the lax posterior capsule stretches over time on weight-bearing.
- In knees with varus > recurvatum deformity, correction of varus deformity will increase the extension gap; hence, distal femur cut should be decreased by 2 mm or more.

Varus ≈ Recurvatum

- The full-length radiographs of the lower limb with AP and lateral views of the right knee (**Fig. 3.51**).
- X-rays demonstrate tricompartmental osteoarthritis with varus deformity.
- The navigation kinematic analysis of this patient elicits an equal measure of varus and recurvatum deformity (**Fig. 3.52**).
- There is gradual correction of the varus deformity beyond 60 degrees of knee flexion.
- The dynamic nature of the coronal plane deformity suggests that the medial soft tissues are lax in knee flexion. Hence, minimal soft tissue release is required to balance the knee.
- Undersection of distal femur was performed considering hyperextension and eroded cartilage (**Fig. 3.53**).
- An image depicting the resected distal femur with eroded articular cartilage over the medial femoral condyle (**Fig. 3.54**).
- The navigation values demonstrate under-resection of the tibial cut (**Fig. 3.55**).
- An image showing the resected proximal tibia with eroded articular cartilage and minimal bone resected from the medial tibial plateau (**Fig. 3.56**).
- A medial osteophyte may be hidden beneath the MCL (**Fig. 3.57**).
- A small osteotome can be used to excise it.
- This decreases the tenting of the MCL fibers and relaxes the medial joint space without requiring any further soft tissue release.
- There is complete correction of deformity, both in sagittal and coronal planes, with the residual flexion of 5 degrees (**Fig. 3.58**).
- The postoperative AP and lateral X-ray views of the knee showing well-placed femoral and tibial components (**Fig. 3.59**).

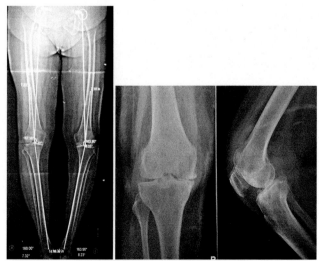

Fig. 3.51 Preoperative radiographs.

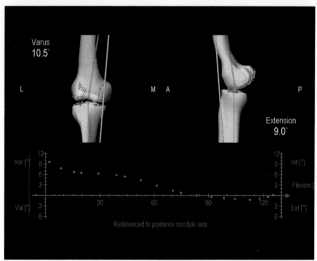

Fig. 3.52 Initial limb alignment and kinematics.

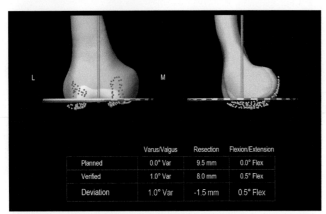

	Varus/Valgus	Resection	Flexion/Extension
Planned	0.0° Var	9.5 mm	0.0° Flex
Verified	1.0° Var	8.0 mm	0.5° Flex
Deviation	1.0° Var	-1.5 mm	0.5° Flex

Fig. 3.53 Conservative distal femur resection.

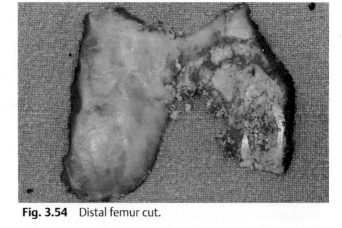

Fig. 3.54 Distal femur cut.

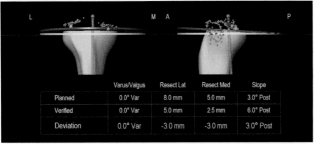

	Varus/Valgus	Resect Lat	Resect Med	Slope
Planned	0.0° Var	8.0 mm	5.0 mm	3.0° Post
Verified	0.0° Var	5.0 mm	2.5 mm	6.0° Post
Deviation	0.0° Var	-3.0 mm	-3.0 mm	3.0° Post

Fig. 3.55 Proximal tibia cut verification.

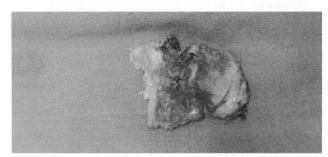

Fig. 3.56 Proximal tibia cut.

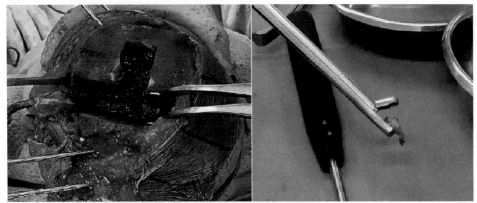

Fig. 3.57 Medial osteophyte hidden under MCL origin on medial femoral condyle is removed.

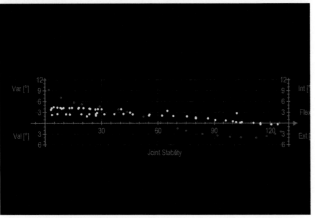

Fig. 3.58 Postoperative limb alignment and kinematics.

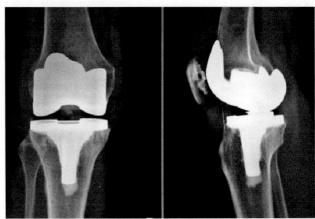

Fig. 3.59 Postoperative radiographs.

Varus < Recurvatum

- The preoperative long-leg radiographs and clinical images depict subluxed tibia along with varus and recurvatum deformity of the left knee (**Fig. 3.60** and **Fig. 3.61**).
- Preoperative kinematics suggest severe varus and hyperextension deformities of left knee with recurvatum (17.5 degrees) > varus (12 degrees) (**Fig. 3.62** and **Fig. 3.63**).
- A 3- to 4-mm under-resection of the distal femur was planned to manage the loose extension gap (**Fig. 3.64**).
- Minimal distal femur cut to balance loose extension gap (**Fig. 3.65**).
- To correct residual varus deformity, tibial tray was downsized from size 3 to 2 (**Fig. 3.66** to **Fig. 3.68**).

- Residual PM bone was marked and removed.
- Tibial baseplate should be at lateral edge of tibia and in external rotation with respect to tibial tuberosity.
- To correct the varus deformity (tight medial gap) PM tibial reduction osteotomy was performed (**Fig. 3.69**).
- The tibial tray was appropriately sized and excess PM bone was marked.
- A saw can be used to remove residual medial bone to open up the tight medial space and correct residual varus.
- The final kinematic analysis showing correction of the varus and hyperextension deformities (**Fig. 3.70**).
- The postoperative radiographs showing well-aligned femoral and tibial prosthetic components with a 3 to 5 degrees of residual flexion, which is desirable in patients with recurvatum deformity (**Fig. 3.71**).

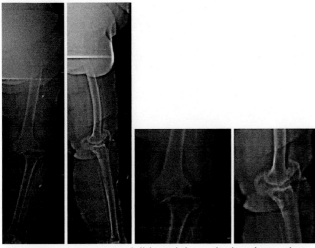

Fig. 3.60 Preoperative full-length lower limb radiographs.

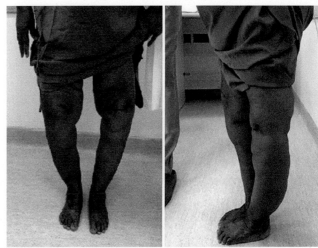

Fig. 3.61 Preop image of the patient.

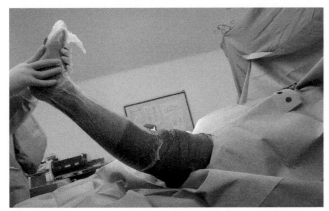

Fig. 3.62 Severe recurvatum deformity after anesthesia.

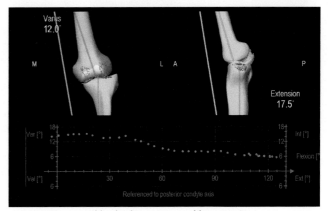

Fig. 3.63 Initial limb alignment and kinematics.

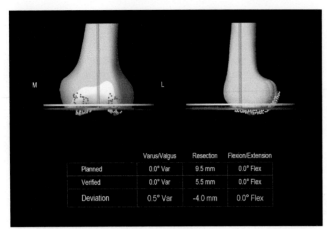

Fig. 3.64 Distal femur cut verification.

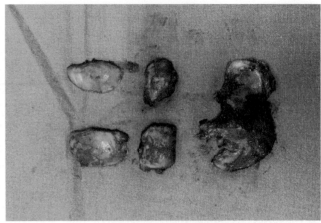

Fig. 3.65 Conservative distal femur and proximal tibia cut.

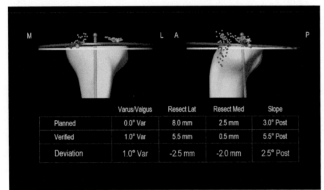

Fig. 3.66 Proximal tibia cut verification.

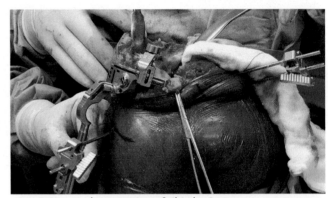

Fig. 3.67 Under resection of tibia by 2 mm.

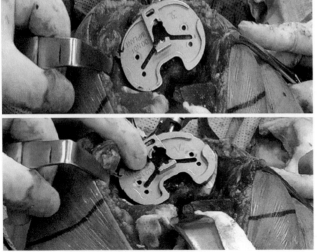

Fig. 3.68 Downsizing of tibial baseplate.

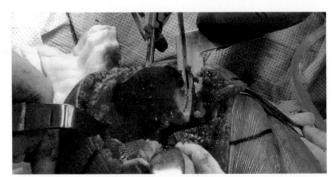

Fig. 3.69 Reduction osteotomy of tibia.

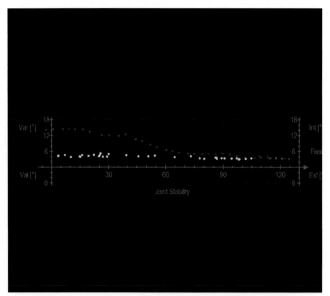

Fig. 3.70 Postoperative limb alignment and kinematics.

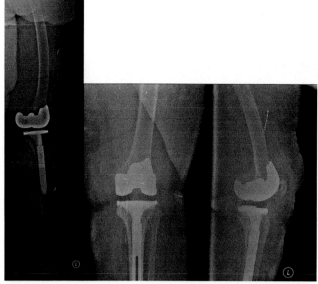

Fig. 3.71 Postoperative radiographs.

Varus > Recurvatum

- The preoperative radiographs show a subluxed tibia with severe varus deformity (**Fig. 3.72**).
- There is 15-degree uncorrectable varus deformity with 5-degree recurvatum (**Fig. 3.73**).
- The navigation values reveal an under-resection of the distal femur (1–2 mm) to compensate for the loose extension gap following varus correction (**Fig. 3.74**).
- The navigation values demonstrate less than normal proximal tibial cut (**Fig. 3.75**).
- This was done as the patient had a loose extension gap along with an equally lax flexion space.
- Severe varus was corrected by tibia reduction osteotomy and posteromedial soft tissue release.
- A screw was used for the residual medial tibial condyle bone defect (**Fig. 3.76**).

Pearls

The authors prefer the following for managing tibial condyle bone defects:
- 0- to 5-mm defect—cement only.
- 5 to 10 mm—augmentation with screw.
- >10 mm—bone graft and tibial extension rod.

- It is advisable to leave these patients in 5 to 7 degrees of residual flexion to prevent recurrence of recurvatum postoperatively (**Fig. 3.77**).
- The postoperative radiographs suggesting well-aligned femoral and tibial components with a screw in the medial tibial condyle to compensate for the residual bone defect (**Fig. 3.78**).

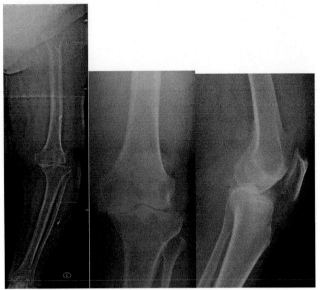

Fig. 3.72 Preoperative radiographs.

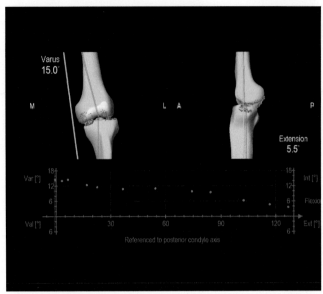

Fig. 3.73 Initial limb alignment and kinematics.

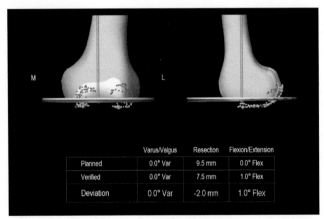

Fig. 3.74 Distal femur cut verification.

	Varus/Valgus	Resection	Flexion/Extension
Planned	0.0° Var	9.5 mm	0.0° Flex
Verified	0.0° Var	7.5 mm	1.0° Flex
Deviation	0.0° Var	-2.0 mm	1.0° Flex

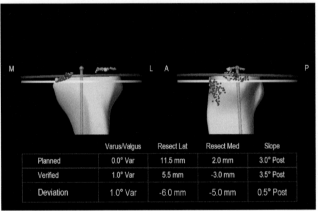

Fig. 3.75 Proximal tibia cut verification.

	Varus/Valgus	Resect Lat	Resect Med	Slope
Planned	0.0° Var	11.5 mm	2.0 mm	3.0° Post
Verified	1.0° Var	5.5 mm	-3.0 mm	3.5° Post
Deviation	1.0° Var	-6.0 mm	-5.0 mm	0.5° Post

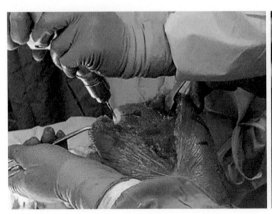

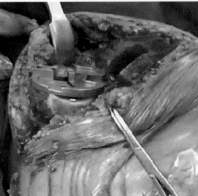

Fig. 3.76 Screw fixation for bone defect.

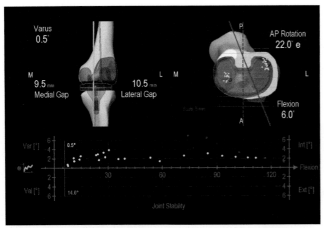

Fig. 3.77 Postoperative limb alignment and kinematics.

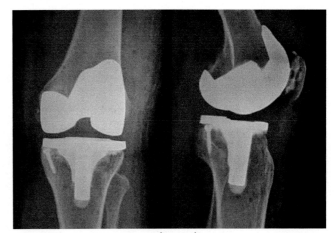

Fig. 3.78 Postoperative radiographs.

Points to Remember

- Varus is often associated with flexion deformity. If varus is near equal to flexion deformity, correction of varus corrects FFD roughly in 1:1 ratio. In such cases soft tissue releases are done to correct varus which also results in correction of FFD.
- If FFD > varus, then additional distal femur bone cut may be required along with soft tissue releases to correct FFD so as to achieve neutral alignment in coronal and sagittal planes.
- If varus is more than FFD, then correction of varus may lead to increase in extension gap and extension laxity; hence, distal femur cut can be conservative especially in severe varus deformity.
- Similarly, varus is sometimes associated with recurvatum deformity. These represent a variety of lax knees with loose gaps. Both distal femur and tibia cut need to be conservative when varus is near equal to recurvatum.
- When varus is more than recurvatum, correction of varus deformity will increase the extension space and hence distal femur cut needs to be conservative to prevent recurrence of recurvatum.
- When recurvatum is more than varus, extreme caution needs to be exercised as these knees are most prone to recurrence of hyperextension deformity. Along with conservative cuts and minimal handling of soft tissues, a constrained poly can be used to attain stability.

References

1. Sharma L, Song J, Dunlop D, et al. Varus and valgus alignment and incident and progressive knee osteoarthritis. Ann Rheum Dis 2010;69(11):1940–1945

2. Goulston LM, Sanchez-Santos MT, D'Angelo S, et al. A comparison of radiographic anatomic axis knee alignment measurements and cross-sectional associations with knee osteoarthritis. Osteoarthritis Cartilage 2016;24(4):612–622

3. Xiao-Gang Z, Shahzad K, Li C. One-stage total knee arthroplasty for patients with osteoarthritis of the knee and extra-articular deformity. Int Orthop 2012;36(12):2457–2463

4. Moon YW, Kim JG, Han JH, Do KH, Seo JG, Lim HC. Factors correlated with the reducibility of varus deformity in knee osteoarthritis: an analysis using navigation guided TKA. Clin Orthop Surg 2013;5(1):36–43

5. Buza JA III, Wasterlain AS, Thakkar SC, Meere P, Vigdorchik J. Navigation and robotics in knee arthroplasty. JBJS Rev 2017;5(2)

6. Yasgur DJ, Scuderi GR, Insall JN. Medial release for fixed varus deformity surgical techniques. In: Scuderi GR, Tria AJ, eds. Total knee arthroplasty. New York: Springer; 2002:189–196

7. Verdonk PC, Pernin J, Pinaroli A, Ait Si Selmi T, Neyret P. Soft tissue balancing in varus total knee arthroplasty: an algorithmic approach. Knee Surg Sports Traumatol Arthrosc 2009;17(6):660–666

8. Dixon MC, Parsch D, Brown RR, Scott RD. The correction of severe varus deformity in total knee arthroplasty by tibial component downsizing and resection of uncapped proximal medial bone. J Arthroplasty 2004;19(1):19–22

9. Mullaji AB, Shetty GM. Surgical technique: Computer-assisted sliding medial condylar osteotomy to achieve gap balance in varus knees during TKA. Clin Orthop Relat Res 2013;471(5):1484–1491

Computer-Navigated TKR for Valgus and Associated Sagittal Deformities

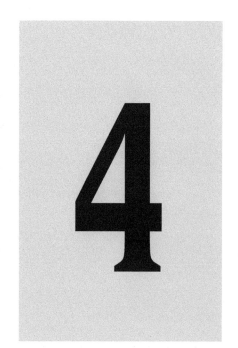

Anoop Jhurani and Piyush Agarwal

Introduction

- 10 to 12% of all patients undergoing primary total knee arthroplasty (TKA) present with a valgus deformity.[1]
- Valgus deformity differs from varus in three principal ways:
  - Valgus originates primarily from femur whereas the varus deformity comes from the tibia.[2]
  - Valgus knee is loose in flexion and there is a hypoplasia of lateral femoral condyle distally and posteriorly.[3]
  - Valgus may be associated with an inflammatory pathology like rheumatoid arthritis or with skeletal development anomalies like genu valgum.[4]
- Other causes of valgus deformity are primary osteoarthritis, posttraumatic arthritis, and overcorrection of proximal tibial osteotomy.[5]
- In comparison to varus deformity, valgus deformity has its own set of perioperative challenges[4–6]:
  - Lateral bone loss in the femur and/or tibia.
  - Metaphyseal remodeling of femur and tibia.
  - External rotational deformity of the distal femur.
  - Patellar maltracking or subluxation.
  - Contracture of lateral soft tissues.
  - Laxity of the medial ligamentous structures.

- Severe valgus knees are generally associated with poorer outcomes when matched to severe varus knees.[7]
- It is difficult to estimate the orientation of the distal femur cut by conventional method in valgus deformity. Literature varies in its recommendation from 3 to 5 degrees of femur valgus, while performing distal femur cut.[4]
- Computer navigation helps assess and quantify the deformity in a valgus knee.[8]
- In cases of rigid valgus deformity, navigation proves to be a valuable tool to perform soft tissue releases or a lateral epicondylar osteotomy.[9]
- Similar to the varus knees, valgus presents mostly a biplanar deformity. Therefore, the correction of a coronal plane deformity should be closely evaluated in association with a sagittal plane deformity.
- To simplify, valgus knees can be divided into:
  - Valgus associated with a fixed flexion deformity (FFD):
    - Valgus ≈ FFD.
    - Valgus < FFD.
    - Valgus > FFD.
  - Valgus associated with a recurvatum deformity:
    - Valgus ≈ Recurvatum.
    - Valgus < Recurvatum.
    - Valgus > Recurvatum.

Principles

- The femur has valgus remodeling in most cases and navigation assists in executing an accurate distal femur cut. The distal femur cut can be kept in 1 to 2 degree varus to help correct overall limb alignment.
- The posterior condylar axis should not be used for femoral rotation because of lateral condylar hypoplasia. Navigation helps in predicting femoral component rotation in accordance with the interepicondylar axis.
- The tibia is also remodeled in valgus in most cases. An accurate tibial cut is possible with navigation control.
- Iliotibial (IT) band release is mostly required to correct valgus in extension and popliteus to correct tight lateral flexion gap. The posterolateral capsule is released in extension when valgus is associated with FFD.

Navigation for Valgus Knees with Flexion Deformity

- Valgus knees are generally associated with a loose flexion gap. The accompanying flexion deformity further makes gap balancing challenging in such knees.[3]
- Navigation accurately predicts the medial and lateral gaps at different knee range which guides the surgeon for soft tissue releases required to achieve a balanced knee.

Algorithm for Planning Distal Femur Resection in Valgus Knee with Fixed Flexion Deformity

- In a uniplanar valgus deformity, a normal distal femur cut would result in an adequate extension gap post deformity correction.
- In knees with a valgus and fixed flexion deformity, an additional distal femur resection is recommended to compensate for the tight extension gap.
- Valgus deformity associated with an FFD can be divided in the following categories:
    - Valgus ≈ FFD.
    - Valgus > FFD.
    - Valgus < FFD.

Valgus = FFD

- The preoperative X-rays and the clinical images show a mild valgus with flexion deformity (**Fig. 4.1** and **Fig. 4.2**).
- No significant posterior osteophytes are seen in the lateral view.
- The preoperative navigation kinematics demonstrated an equal coronal (10.5 degrees) and sagittal plane deformity (9 degrees) with the knee reaching a neutral alignment at 90-degree flexion (**Fig. 4.3**).
- An additional distal femur resection was required to balance the tight extension gap (**Fig. 4.4** and **Fig. 4.5**).
- A measured proximal tibial resection was done with navigation (**Fig. 4.6** and **Fig. 4.7**).

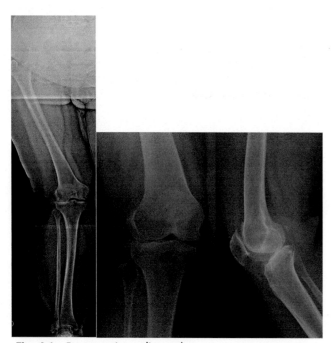

Fig. 4.1 Preoperative radiographs.

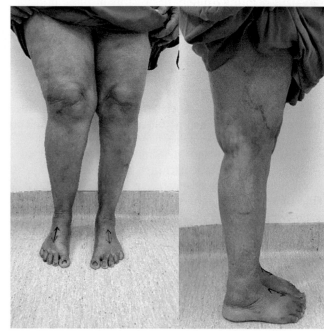

Fig. 4.2 Frontal and side views of the patient.

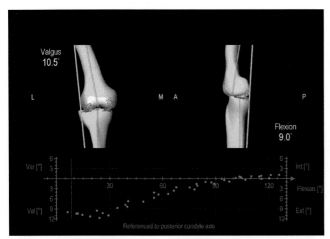

Fig. 4.3 Initial limb alignment and deformity.

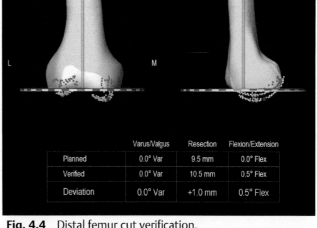

	Varus/Valgus	Resection	Flexion/Extension
Planned	0.0° Var	9.5 mm	0.0° Flex
Verified	0.0° Var	10.5 mm	0.5° Flex
Deviation	0.0° Var	+1.0 mm	0.5° Flex

Fig. 4.4 Distal femur cut verification.

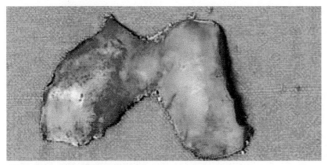

Fig. 4.5 Distal femur cut.

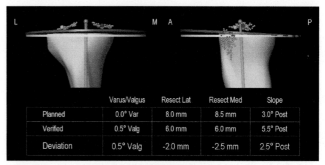

	Varus/Valgus	Resect Lat	Resect Med	Slope
Planned	0.0° Var	8.0 mm	8.5 mm	3.0° Post
Verified	0.5° Valg	6.0 mm	6.0 mm	5.5° Post
Deviation	0.5° Valg	-2.0 mm	-2.5 mm	2.5° Post

Fig. 4.6 Proximal tibia cut verification.

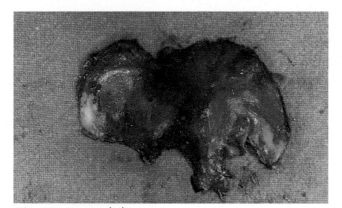

Fig. 4.7 Proximal tibia cut.

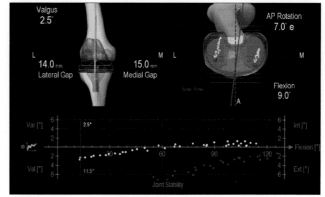

Fig. 4.8 Limb alignment before soft tissue releases.

- In this patient, an underresection of -2mm was planned for the tibia.
- Bony cuts and soft tissue balance can be verified with the help of navigation.
- Navigation can be used to identify residual deformity with trials (**Fig. 4.8**).
- Distal femur cut should be in 0.5- to 1-degree varus to aid in overall correction of deformity.

- Tibial cut can be in 0.5- to 1.5-degree varus, with 6 to 8 mm thickness.
- Rotation should be set parallel to the interepicondylar axis.
- IT band may need pie crusting in extension to correct valgus deformity and popliteus may require pie crusting to open up the tight lateral flexion space.

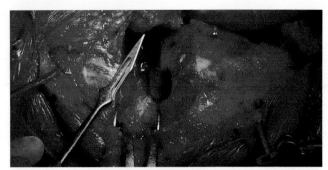

Fig. 4.9 11# blade for pie crusting of iliotibial (IT) band.

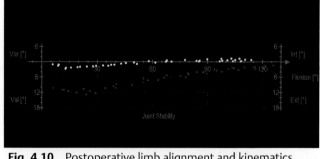

Fig. 4.10 Postoperative limb alignment and kinematics.

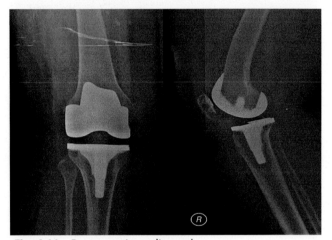

Fig. 4.11 Postoperative radiographs.

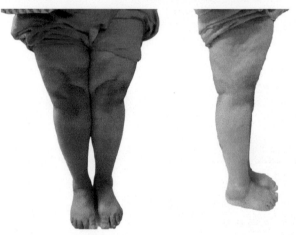

Fig. 4.12 Coronal and sagittal alignment at the end of 2 years.

Pearls

- The authors prefer to use the tip of a #11 blade for pie crusting of the IT band (**Fig. 4.9**).
- The soft tissue releases are titrated under navigation control till neutral alignment is achieved. This prevents over release and instability.

- The postoperative kinematic analysis demonstrates the complete correction of the biplanar deformity (**Fig. 4.10**).
- The postoperative radiographs demonstrated satisfactory prosthesis position and alignment (**Fig. 4.11**).
- Postoperative coronal and sagittal alignment at 2 year of follow-up (**Fig. 4.12**).

Valgus > Flexion Deformity

- The preoperative radiographs and the clinical image reveal a moderate valgus deformity (11 degrees) associated with flexion deformity (5 degrees) (**Fig. 4.13** and **Fig. 4.14**).
- The preoperative kinematic analysis suggests a moderate valgus deformity, gradually correcting with progressive knee flexion (**Fig. 4.15**).
- The soft tissue behavior can be depicted from this kinematic analysis.
- The patient may require a popliteus pie crust to balance the tight lateral gap in flexion.
- The intraoperative clinical images show a contained defect in the lateral tibial condyle (**Fig. 4.16**).
- Distal femoral cut (DFC) in valgus knees can be taken in 0.5- to 1.5-degree varus to compensate for the valgus present in the distal femur and to keep the overall alignment in varus (**Fig. 4.17**).
- Navigation accurately predicted the thickness of the medial and lateral tibial condyle cuts (**Fig. 4.18**).

- As with the DFC, a varus cut of 0.5 to 1 degree can be taken in the proximal tibia to compensate for the valgus tibial deformity.
- Popliteus tendon pie crusting for the tight lateral gap in flexion (**Fig. 4.19**).

Pearls

- The authors prefer pie crusting over the complete release of the popliteus tendon.
- A 21-gauge needle is used for pie crusting which relaxes the tight fibers of the popliteus tendon without hampering its function.
- A complete release of the tendon is reserved for severe deformities.

- The postoperative kinematic analysis demonstrated the correction of the valgus deformity throughout the knee ROM (**Fig. 4.20**).

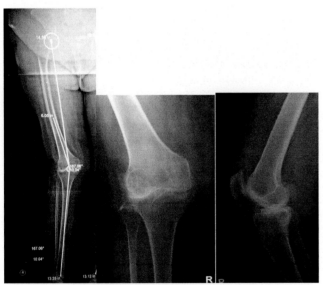

Fig. 4.13 Preoperative radiographs.

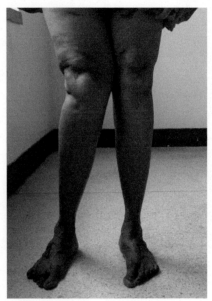

Fig. 4.14 Preoperative image of the patient.

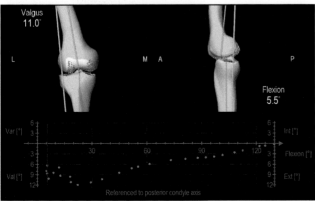

Fig. 4.15 Initial limb alignment and kinematics.

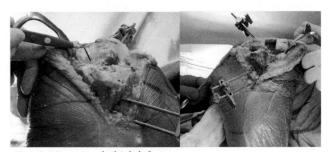

Fig. 4.16 Lateral tibial defect.

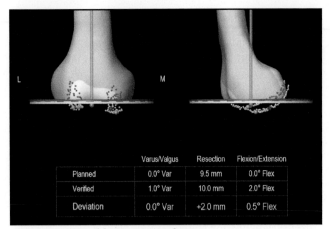

	Varus/Valgus	Resection	Flexion/Extension
Planned	0.0° Var	9.5 mm	0.0° Flex
Verified	1.0° Var	10.0 mm	2.0° Flex
Deviation	0.0° Var	+2.0 mm	0.5° Flex

Fig. 4.17 Distal femur cut verification.

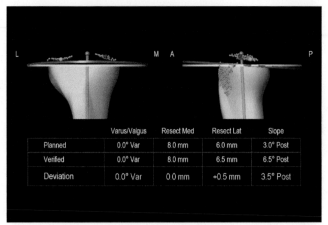

	Varus/Valgus	Resect Med	Resect Lat	Slope
Planned	0.0° Var	8.0 mm	6.0 mm	3.0° Post
Verified	0.0° Var	8.0 mm	6.5 mm	6.5° Post
Deviation	0.0° Var	0.0 mm	+0.5 mm	3.5° Post

Fig. 4.18 Proximal tibial cut verification.

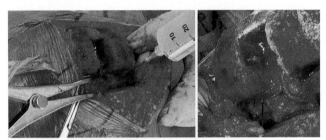

Fig. 4.19 Popliteus tendon pie crusting.

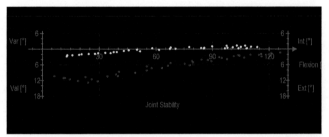

Fig. 4.20 Postoperative limb alignment and kinematics.

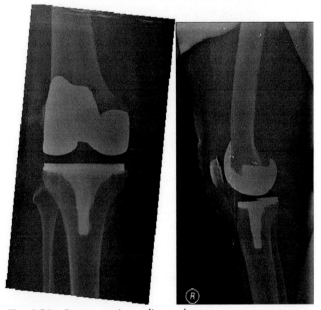

Fig. 4.21 Postoperative radiographs.

- The postoperative X-rays shows well-aligned tibial and femoral prosthetic components (**Fig. 4.21**).

Pitfalls

The correction of a severe valgus deformity may lead to common peroneal nerve (CPN) injury.

- A large thickness insert could lead to a traction-type injury to the CPN. A conservative tibial cut and continuous assessment of gaps during surgery is recommended to prevent large gaps and inserts. The aim should be to use minimum thickness inserts in most cases.

Valgus < Fixed Flexion Deformity

- The preoperative radiographs and patient's image show a moderate valgus deformity (**Fig. 4.22** and **Fig. 4.23**).
- The lateral radiograph reveals the posterior osteophytes and advanced patellofemoral arthritis.

- Proximal tibial cut with a decreased posterior slope is advised.
- The preoperative kinematics navigation graph demonstrated an FFD (18.5 degrees) > valgus deformity (11.5 degrees) (**Fig. 4.24**).
- The valgus deformity gradually corrected with progressive knee flexion.
- An additional 3 mm of distal femur cut was planned to balance the loose flexion gap associated with the valgus knee (**Fig. 4.25**).
- Caution should be exercised to prevent damage to the attachments of the collateral ligaments while executing + 2 to 3 distal femur cut.
- The DFC was kept in 0.5-degree varus to maintain a neutral to varus overall limb alignment postoperatively.

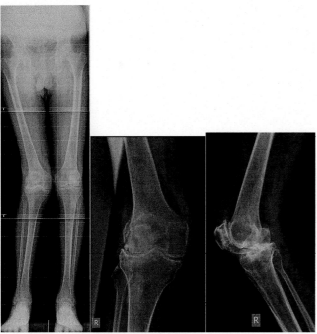

Fig. 4.22 Preoperative radiographs.

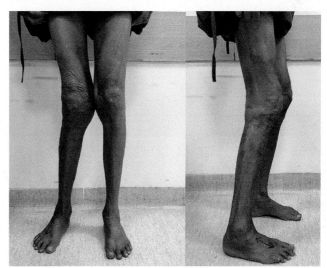

Fig. 4.23 Preoperative image of the patient.

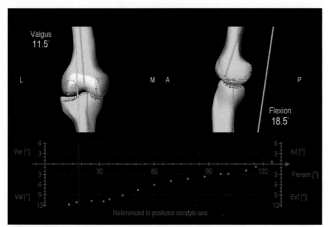

Fig. 4.24 Initial limb alignment and kinematics.

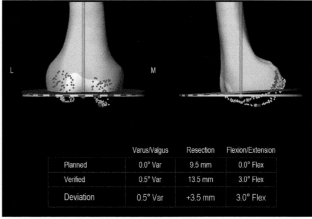

Fig. 4.25 Distal femur cut verification.

	Varus/Valgus	Resection	Flexion/Extension
Planned	0.0° Var	9.5 mm	0.0° Flex
Verified	0.5° Var	13.5 mm	3.0° Flex
Deviation	0.5° Var	+3.5 mm	3.0° Flex

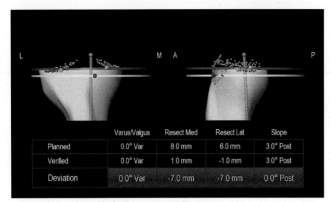

Fig. 4.26 Proximal tibia cut verification.

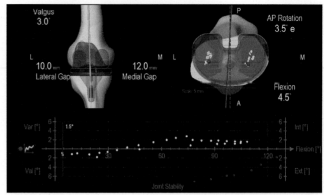

Fig. 4.27 Limb alignment before soft tissue releases.

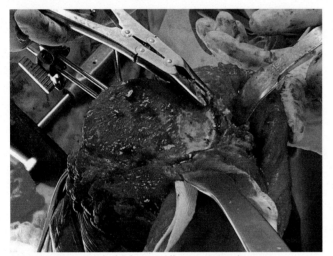

Fig. 4.28 Lateral tibial osteophytes removal.

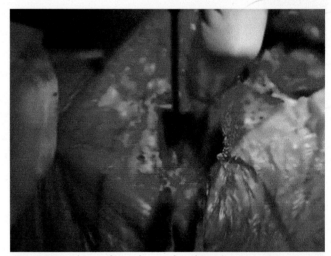

Fig. 4.29 Posterolateral capsule release in extension.

- A varus tibial cut in a varus knee and a valgus tibial cut in a valgus knee is a common intraoperative error that can lead to early prosthesis failure (**Fig. 4.26**).
- The navigation-assisted verification of the proximal tibial cut can identify the error and help the surgeon to rectify it.
- An under-resection of the proximal tibia was planned to manage the gaps with a 9 mm insert.
- Navigation is used for predicting residual deformity with trials, and soft tissue release can be titrated accordingly (**Fig. 4.27**).
- Removal of lateral tibial osteophytes relaxes lateral soft tissues (**Fig. 4.28**).
- This increases extension and corrects mediolateral gap imbalance.
- The lateral osteophytes should be excised before tibial tray sizing.
- The posterolateral osteophytes may lead to flexion deformity and oversizing of the tibia tray.
- A 10-mm curved osteotome is preferred to remove the osteophytes.

- The posterolateral neurovasculature structures are in close association with the osteophytes. Caution must be exerted while removing them.
- A clinical picture depicting the posterolateral capsular release (**Fig. 4.29**).
- The posterolateral capsular release is performed with the electrocautery in full extension.
- A laminar spreader is placed on the medial side.
- The authors use a long-tip electrocautery and a 20-mm osteotome as a guide for capsular release.

Pitfalls

The surgeon should be aware of the potential risks of thermal injury to the common perineal nerve with the usage of the cautery. The nerve lies 1.5- to 2-cm posterolateral to the popliteus tendon.

- The complete correction of the biplanar deformity in the postoperative kinematics graph (**Fig. 4.30**).

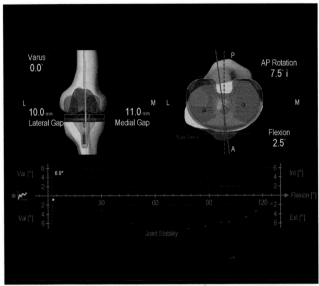

Fig. 4.30 Postoperative limb alignment and kinematics.

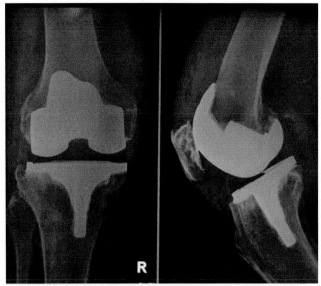

Fig. 4.31 Postoperative radiographs.

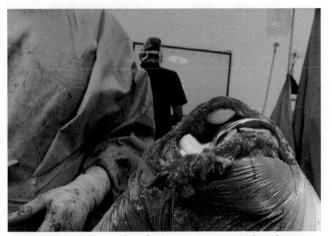

Fig. 4.32 Patellar maltracking is common in valgus knees.

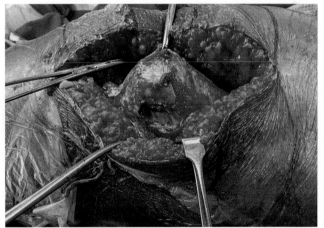

Fig. 4.33 Outside-in lateral retinaculum release.

- Well-aligned tibiofemoral components are seen in postoperative radiographs (**Fig. 4.31**).

Patellar Tracking

- The postoperative image reveals maltracking of the patellar component (**Fig. 4.32**).
- Tracking should be checked without external support of a thumb or a clamp.
- Complications as a result of patellar maltracking include:
  - Chronic pain (anterior knee pain).
  - Decreased ROM.
  - Increased risk of lateral patellar subluxation or dislocation.
- A clinical picture showing the outside-in technique for release of the lateral retinaculum for improved patellar tracking (**Fig. 4.33**).[10]

Pearls

- This technique leaves the synovium intact laterally, decreasing the extravasation of blood in the subcutaneous plane.
- This keeps the joint cavity intact, potentially decreasing the risk of postoperative infections.

Technique

- The lateral skin flap is raised to expose the lateral retinaculum.
- The release is started 1 cm lateral to the lateral border of the patella.
- The direction of release is from distal to proximal, from upper tibial border to midpatella level.

- Superolateral genicular artery should be cauterized if release needs to be extended superiorly.
- Clinical picture showing satisfactory patellar tracking without any external support (**Fig. 4.34**).

Navigation for Valgus with Hyperextension Deformity

- Hyperextension associated with valgus deformity can be missed until carefully looked for.
- Such biplanar deformities result in loose flexion and extension gaps due to lax tissues and joint capsule, making gap balancing critical.
- A normal DFC is planned to compensate for the loose flexion space.
- A conservative tibial cut is planned to balance the gaps with a minimal thickness insert.

Algorithm for Planning Distal Femur Resection in Valgus Deformity with Recurvatum

- In knees with a valgus and recurvatum deformity, normal or near-normal DFC (according to the implant thickness) needs to be taken to prevent a postoperative flexion deformity.
- The DFC is decreased only in cases with severe joint laxity or with recurvatum > 10 degrees. For such lax knees, a constrained prosthesis should be available.
- To prevent the usage of thicker inserts, a conservative tibial cut should be taken.
- Valgus deformity associated with recurvatum deformity can be divided in the following categories.
  - Valgus ≈ Recurvatum.
  - Valgus > Recurvatum.
  - Valgus < Recurvatum.

Valgus ≈ Recurvatum

- The preoperative radiographs reveal a mild valgus deformity. It is worthy to note valgoid tibial remodeling present in most valgus cases (**Fig. 4.35**).
- The lateral view shows neutral slope on tibia which is a common finding in knees with recurvatum.
- The preoperative kinematics graph demonstrated an equal valgus (6.5 degrees) and recurvatum deformity (6 degrees) (**Fig. 4.36**).
- 9.5-mm distal femur cut to compensate for the loose flexion gap (**Fig. 4.37**).

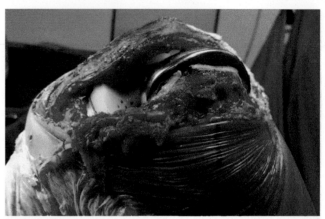

Fig. 4.34 Patella in complete contact with the medial condyle of the femoral component after "outside-in" release.

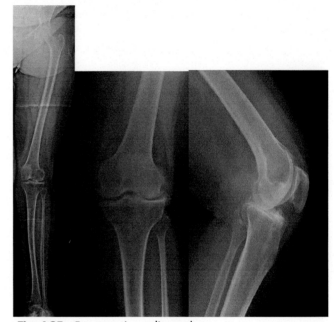

Fig. 4.35 Preoperative radiographs.

- The femoral component rotation was increased to compensate for the lateral femoral condyle hypoplasia[11] (**Fig. 4.38** and **Fig. 4.39**).
- An internal rotation or decreased external rotation of the femoral component may lead to complications such as gap imbalance or patellar maltracking.
- This instrument is placed on pins for anteroposterior (AP) cutter jig to manually check rotation of femoral component in alliance to transepidcondylar axis and Whiteside line[12] (**Fig. 4.40**).
- The navigation values demonstrate a conservative tibial cut as both the flexion and extension gaps were loose (**Fig. 4.41**).
- The proximal tibia resection referencing is done from the bony defect in the lateral tibial condyle with the cut thickness measured at 0 to 2 mm from the base of the defect (**Fig. 4.42**).

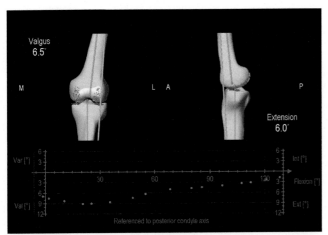

Fig. 4.36 Initial limb alignment and kinematics.

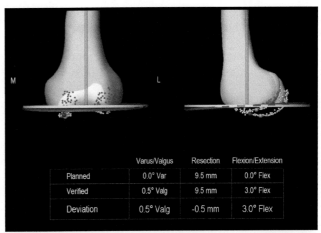

Fig. 4.37 Distal femur cut verification.

	Varus/Valgus	Resection	Flexion/Extension
Planned	0.0° Var	9.5 mm	0.0° Flex
Verified	0.5° Valg	9.5 mm	3.0° Flex
Deviation	0.5° Valg	-0.5 mm	3.0° Flex

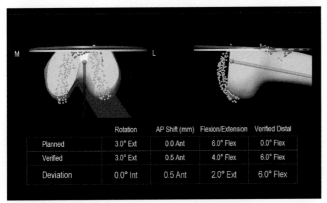

Fig. 4.38 Femoral external rotation verification.

	Rotation	AP Shift (mm)	Flexion/Extension	Verified Distal
Planned	3.0° Ext	0.0 Ant	6.0° Flex	0.0° Flex
Verified	3.0° Ext	0.5 Ant	4.0° Flex	6.0° Flex
Deviation	0.0° Int	0.5 Ant	2.0° Ext	6.0° Flex

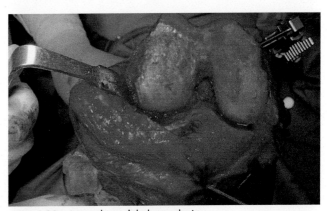

Fig. 4.39 Lateral condyle hypoplasia.

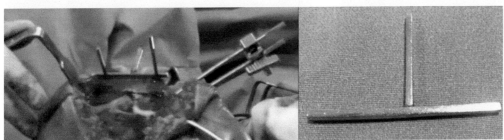

Fig. 4.40 Femoral external rotation verification.

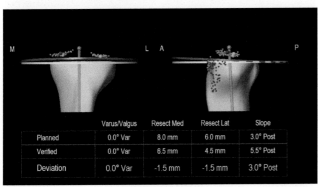

Fig. 4.41 Proximal tibia cut verification.

	Varus/Valgus	Resect Med	Resect Lat	Slope
Planned	0.0° Var	8.0 mm	6.0 mm	3.0° Post
Verified	0.0° Var	6.5 mm	4.5 mm	5.5° Post
Deviation	0.0° Var	-1.5 mm	-1.5 mm	3.0° Post

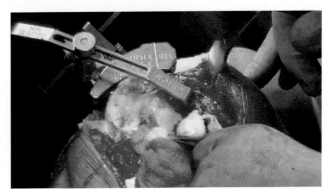

Fig. 4.42 Manual tibial cut thickness verification from lateral tibial condyle defect.

- The final kinematic analysis showing complete correction of the valgus and hyperextension deformities (**Fig. 4.43**).
- The final postoperative radiographs demonstrate well-aligned femoral and tibial components (**Fig. 4.44**).
- Midflexion laxity in severe valgus knees may lead to gap imbalance (**Fig. 4.45**).

- In such cases, there may be mediolateral gap imbalance in spite of all requisite soft tissue releases on lateral side.
- Mediolateral gap imbalance may lead to subluxation or instability (**Fig. 4.46**).
- Semiconstrained insert with broad cam and elevated anterior lip can be used in moderate form of gap imbalance (**Fig. 4.47** and **Fig. 4.48**).

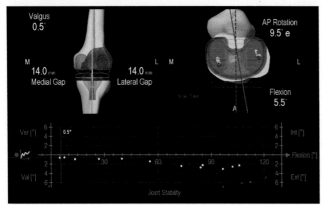

Fig. 4.43 Postoperative limb alignment and kinematics.

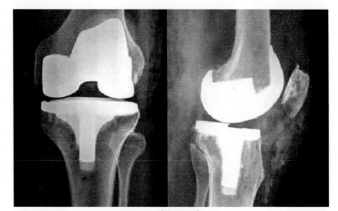

Fig. 4.44 Postoperative radiographs.

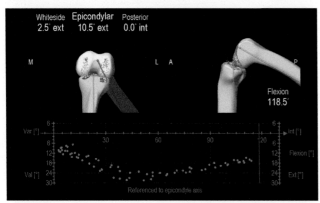

Fig. 4.45 Initial limb alignment and kinematics.

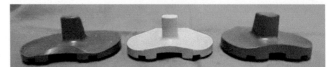

Fig. 4.47 Normal and constrained insert trial.

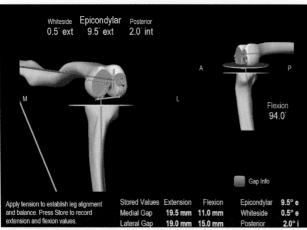

Fig. 4.46 Unbalanced mediolateral gap after cuts and soft tissue releases.

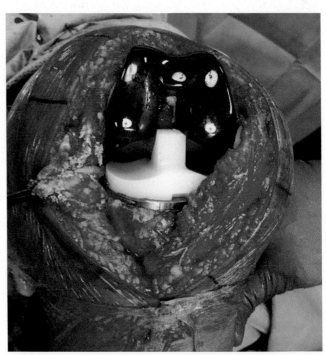

Fig. 4.48 Final total knee arthroplasty (TKA) component with semiconstrained insert.

Valgus > Recurvatum

- The preoperative radiographs show a significant valgus deformity in the left knee with a bipolar prosthesis in the ipsilateral hip (**Fig. 4.49**).
- The advantages of a full-length lower limb X-ray are that it can reveal extra-articular deformity, implant in the proximal or distal joint, femoral shaft bowing, and the overall alignment of the lower limb.
- A significant valgus deformity with mild recurvatum at the left knee joint (**Fig. 4.50**).
- The navigation graph demonstrated 18 degrees of valgus deformity which was corrected with knee flexion, associated with 5.5 degrees of hyperextension in the sagittal plane (**Fig. 4.51**).

Pitfalls

- The complete correction of a severe valgus deformity may lead to a peroneal nerve injury.

- If there are symptoms of a neural injury postoperatively, it is advisable to keep the knee in 30-degree flexion to relax the sciatic nerve.
- Most neural injuries are neuropraxias which may recover within few weeks.

- The navigation software represented an accurate 3D reconstruction of the distal femur anatomy, revealing the presence of lateral femoral condyle hypoplasia (**Fig. 4.52**).
- A normal DFC was planned to compensate for the loose flexion gap (**Fig. 4.53**).
- The navigation values and the intraoperative clinical picture shows a contained bony defect in the lateral tibial condyle (**Fig. 4.54** and **Fig. 4.55**).
- A minimal thickness (-5.5 mm), neutral proximal tibial cut, with a decreased posterior slope, was planned to achieve a balanced knee (**Fig. 4.56**).
- IT band pie crusting for residual valgus deformity (**Fig. 4.57**).

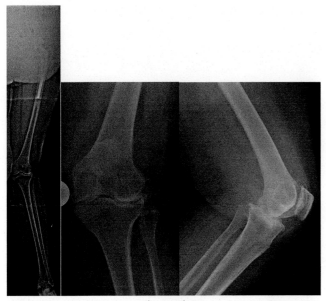

Fig. 4.49　Preoperative radiographs.

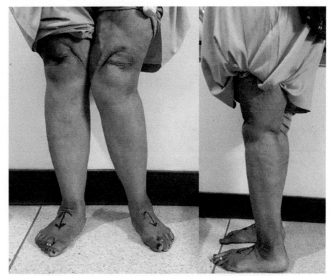

Fig. 4.50　Preoperative image of the patient.

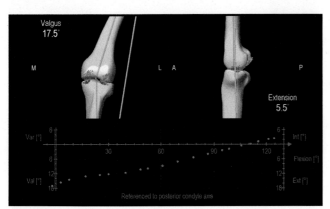

Fig. 4.51　Initial limb alignment and kinematics.

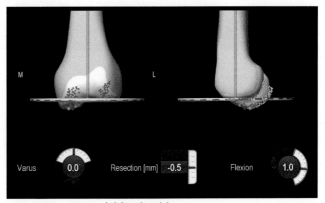

Fig. 4.52　3D model for distal femur.

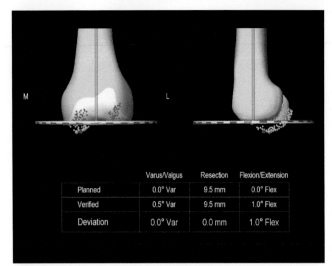

Fig. 4.53 Distal femur cut verification.

	Varus/Valgus	Resection	Flexion/Extension
Planned	0.0° Var	9.5 mm	0.0° Flex
Verified	0.5° Var	9.5 mm	1.0° Flex
Deviation	0.0° Var	0.0 mm	1.0° Flex

- The postoperative kinematic alignment revealed 7 to 8 degrees of sagittal correction with neutral coronal plane alignment (**Fig. 4.58**).
- The postoperative radiographs demonstrate well-aligned knee components with a hip prosthesis on the ipsilateral side (**Fig. 4.59**).

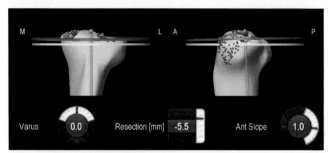

Fig. 4.54 3D model for proximal tibia.

Varus 0.0   Resection [mm] -5.5   Ant Slope 1.0

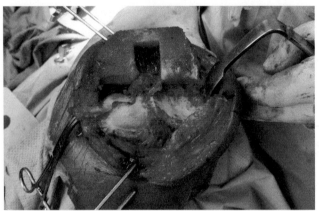

Fig. 4.55 Lateral tibial defect.

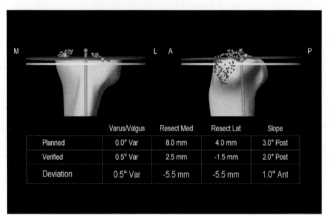

Fig. 4.56 Proximal tibia cut verification.

	Varus/Valgus	Resect Med	Resect Lat	Slope
Planned	0.0° Var	8.0 mm	4.0 mm	3.0° Post
Verified	0.5° Var	2.5 mm	-1.5 mm	2.0° Post
Deviation	0.5° Var	-5.5 mm	-5.5 mm	1.0° Ant

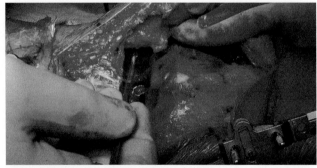

Fig. 4.57 Iliotibial (IT) band pie crusting.

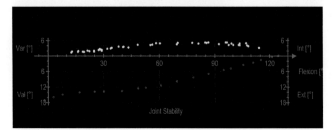

Fig. 4.58 Postoperative limb alignment and kinematics.

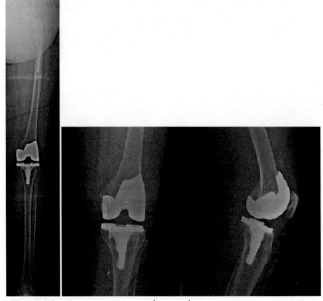

Fig. 4.59 Postoperative radiographs.

Valgus < Recurvatum

- It is of utmost importance to identify this subgroup of patients carefully, as they need under-resection of the distal femur to prevent recurrence of the recurvatum deformity.
- The preoperative radiograph and a clinical picture of the right knee demonstrates a valgus deformity with a laterally subluxed tibia (**Fig. 4.60** and **Fig. 4.61**).
- The preoperative kinematic analysis suggests a significant recurvatum deformity (10.5 degrees) with a valgus deformity (8.5 degrees). A recurvatum of more than 10 degrees is a risk factor to recurrence of recurvatum post-TKA (**Fig. 4.62**).

- Considering a subluxed knee and the associated recurvatum deformity, under-resection of the distal femur by -1.5 mm was performed with the assistance of navigation (**Fig. 4.63** and **Fig. 4.64**).
- 0 to 2 mm of the proximal tibial cut was measured from the lateral tibial condyle defect and an under-resection of the tibia was done with the help of navigation (**Fig. 4.65** to **Fig. 4.67**).
- The postoperative knee kinematics graph demonstrated the complete correction of deformities in both the planes (**Fig. 4.68** and **Fig. 4.69**).

- The postoperative radiographs show well-aligned prosthetic components (**Fig. 4.70**).

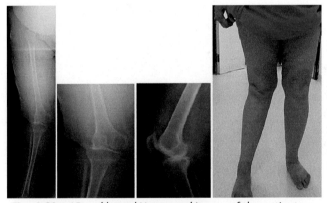

Fig. 4.60 AP and lateral X-rays and image of the patient.

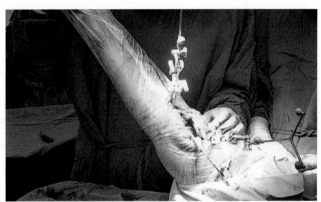

Fig. 4.61 Recurvatum deformity post anesthesia.

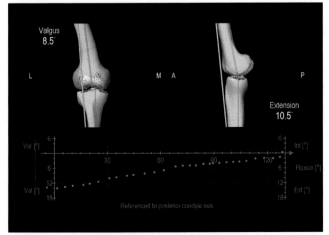

Fig. 4.62 Initial limb alignment and kinematics.

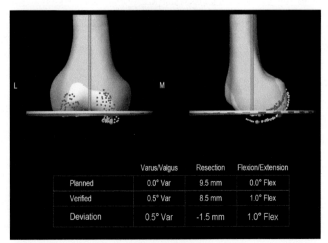

Fig. 4.63 Distal femur cut verification.

	Varus/Valgus	Resection	Flexion/Extension
Planned	0.0° Var	9.5 mm	0.0° Flex
Verified	0.5° Var	8.5 mm	1.0° Flex
Deviation	0.5° Var	-1.5 mm	1.0° Flex

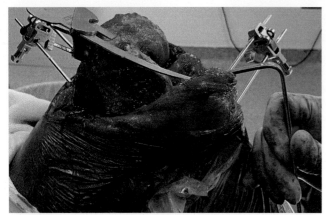

Fig. 4.64 Check by an Angel wing suggesting only medial condyle resection.

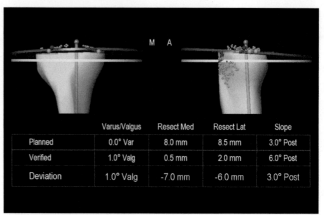

Fig. 4.65 Proximal tibia cut verification.

	Varus/Valgus	Resect Med	Resect Lat	Slope
Planned	0.0° Var	8.0 mm	8.5 mm	3.0° Post
Verified	1.0° Valg	0.5 mm	2.0 mm	6.0° Post
Deviation	1.0° Valg	-7.0 mm	-6.0 mm	3.0° Post

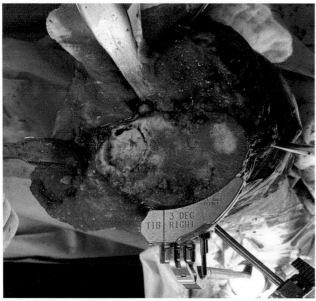

Fig. 4.66 Contained lateral tibial defect after resection.

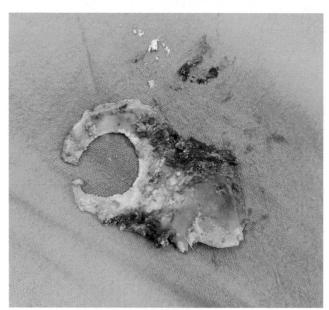

Fig. 4.67 Tibial cut with lateral defect.

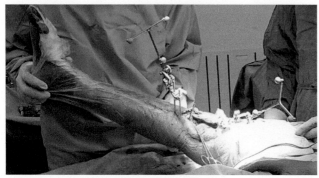

Fig. 4.68 Postoperative sagittal alignment.

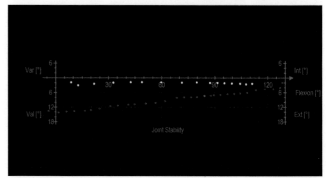

Fig. 4.69 Postoperative limb alignment and kinematics.

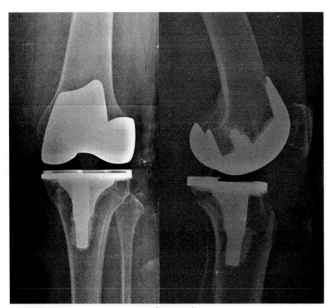

Fig. 4.70 Postoperative radiographs.

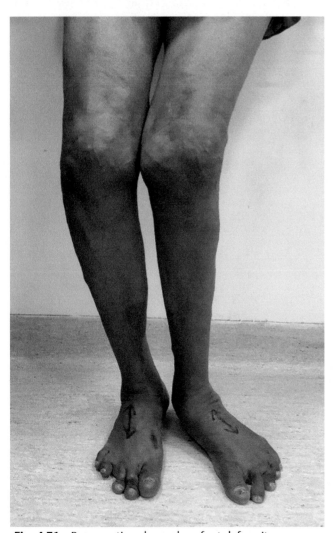

Fig. 4.71 Preoperative planovalgus foot deformity.

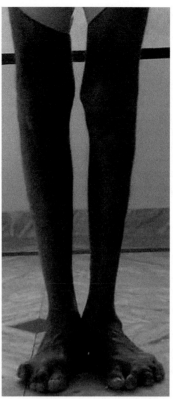

Fig. 4.72 Foot alignment post deformity correction.

Foot Deformity Associated with Valgus Knee

- Foot deformities are commonly associated with severe valgus deformity (**Fig. 4.71**).
- Planovalgus foot deformity causes difficulty in walking and prolonged standing.
- It is advisable to keep such knees in 1 to 3 degrees of varus to compensate for foot malalignment (**Fig. 4.72**).

Points to Remember

- Valgus knees are mostly associated with FFD or recurvatum. Both sets of patients need separate approaches to correct coronal and sagittal plane components of the biplanar deformity.
- The aim is to achieve neutral coronal plane alignment and correct knee to 1 to 3 degree of flexion in valgus knees associated with FFD to prevent recurrence of FFD.
- In knees associated with hyperextension, the aim of sagittal alignment is to keep the knee in 5- to 7-degree flexion to prevent recurrence of recurvatum.
- Both coronal plane correction along with sagittal plane alignment can be achieved predictably with navigation.
- Soft tissue releases in extension and flexion can be guided under navigation to prevent imbalance and instability. However, in severe deformities with mild instability a semiconstrained poly can be used to prevent early failure.

References

1. Ranawat AS, Ranawat CS, Elkus M, Rasquinha VJ, Rossi R, Babhulkar S. Total knee arthroplasty for severe valgus deformity. J Bone Joint Surg Am 2005; 87(Pt 2, Suppl 1):271–284

2. Guo SJ, Zhou YX, Yang DJ, Yang XC. Lower-limb valgus deformity associated with developmental hip dysplasia. Chin Med J (Engl) 2012;125(22):3956–3960

3. Shao JJ, Zhang XL, Wang Q, Chen YS, Shen H, Jiang Y. Total knee arthroplasty using computer assisted navigation in patients with severe valgus deformity of the knee. Chin Med J (Engl) 2010;123(19):2666–2670

4. Nikolopoulos D, Michos I, Safos G, Safos P. Current surgical strategies for total arthroplasty in valgus knee. World J Orthop 2015;6(6):469–482

5. Rossi R, Rosso F, Cottino U, Dettoni F, Bonasia DE, Bruzzone M. Total knee arthroplasty in the valgus knee. Int Orthop 2014; 38(2):273–283

6. Favorito PJ, Mihalko WM, Krackow KA. Total knee arthroplasty in the valgus knee. J Am Acad Orthop Surg 2002;10(1):16–24

7. Karachalios T, Sarangi PP, Newman JH. Severe varus and valgus deformities treated by total knee arthroplasty. J Bone Joint Surg Br 1994;76(6):938–942

8. Huang TW, Lee CY, Lin SJ, et al. Comparison of computer-navigated and conventional total knee arthroplasty in patients with Ranawat type-II valgus deformity: medium-term clinical and radiological results. BMC Musculoskelet Disord 2014;15:390

9. Mullaji AB, Shetty GM. Lateral epicondylar osteotomy using computer navigation in total knee arthroplasty for rigid valgus deformities. J Arthroplasty 2010;25(1):166–169

10. Maniar RN, Singhi T, Rathi SS, Baviskar JV, Nayak RM. Surgical technique: Lateral retinaculum release in knee arthroplasty using a stepwise, outside-in technique. Clin Orthop Relat Res 2012;470(10):2854–2863

11. Mullaji AB, Sharma AK, Marawar SV, Kohli AF, Singh DP. Distal femoral rotational axes in Indian knees. J Orthop Surg (Hong Kong) 2009;17(2):166–169

12. Vanbiervliet J, Bellemans J, Verlinden C, et al. The influence of malrotation and femoral component material on patellofemoral wear during gait. [published correction appears in J Bone Joint Surg Br. 2011 Dec;93(12):1679] J Bone Joint Surg Br 2011;93(10):1348–1354

Computer-Navigated TKR for Fixed Flexion Deformity

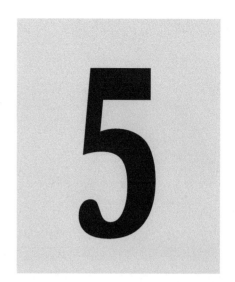

Anoop Jhurani and Piyush Agarwal

Introduction

- Clinical estimation of a fixed flexion deformity (FFD) visually or by a goniometer is likely to be inaccurate.[1]
- The intraoperative estimation of FFD may be fallacious because of obstruction of the anatomical landmarks by surgical drapes and tourniquet.
- With the assistance of computer navigation, this sagittal plane deformity can be diagnosed and quantified precisely.
- Computer navigation can accurately measure the sagittal plane alignment after trials, thereby reducing the probability of a residual fixed flexion or hyperextension postoperatively.
- The presence of an FFD preoperatively is an independent risk factor for developing fixed flexion contracture postoperatively, thus necessitating accurate assessment.[2]
- FFD can be caused by tight posterior capsule, posterior osteophytes, and fibrous adhesions.[3]
- The presence of *bowing in the long bones* of the lower limb may lead to misinterpretation of flexion deformity at the knee clinically. This is particularly valid for the Asian population, who usually have bowing of femur and tibia in both the coronal and sagittal planes, due to childhood Rickets or vit D deficiency.[4]
- Although a flexion deformity in the knee usually presents in association with its coronal counterpart (varus/valgus deformity), this chapter is focused at correction of pure FFD.
- Without the aid of computer navigation, 8 to 17% of patients have risk of postoperative residual FFD.[5,6]

Biomechanics of FFD

- In normal gait pattern, the resultant ground reaction force lies slightly anterior to the center of gravity of knee which helps in maintaining fine balance between hamstrings and quadriceps.
- It allows the knee to lock in extension during stance phase and helps in forward propulsion.
- In knees with FFD, resultant ground reaction force lies posterior to the knee, causing increasing strain over patellofemoral and tibiofemoral joint.
- This causes changes in gait pattern of the patients, making it difficult for them to walk even short distance.
- If FFD is <15 degrees, there is absence of heel strike, with foot placed flat on floor.
- If FFD is >15 degrees, patients walk on toes.
- Other disadvantages of a residual FFD postoperatively:
  - Increased quadriceps activation, resulting in early fatigue.
  - Functional impairment.
  - Limping gait.
  - Problems with activities of daily living.[7]
  - Increased forces across the patellofemoral joint (PFJ) leading to anterior knee pain.[7]
  - Increased stresses at the posterior femoral condyles and posterior tibial plateau on weight-bearing may lead to early failure of the prosthesis.[8]
- Ground reaction force is anterior to the center of the limb in a normal knee. It lies posterior in a knee with FFD (**Fig. 5.1**).

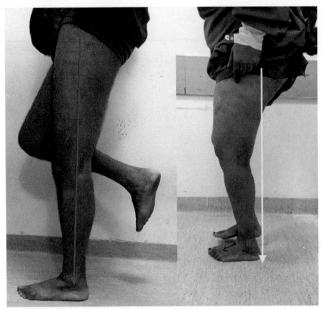

Fig. 5.1 Resultant ground reaction forces in normal knee and knee with fixed flexion deformity (FFD).

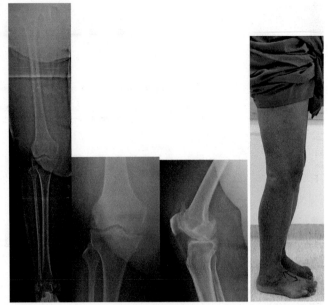

Fig. 5.2 Preoperative radiographs and clinical image of the patient.

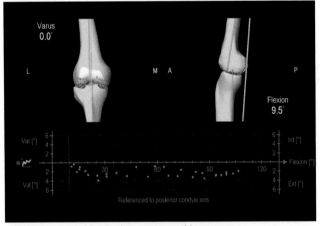

Fig. 5.3 Initial limb alignment and kinematics.

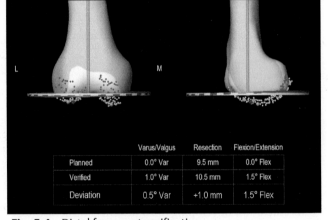

Fig. 5.4 Distal femur cut verification.

	Varus/Valgus	Resection	Flexion/Extension
Planned	0.0° Var	9.5 mm	0.0° Flex
Verified	1.0° Var	10.5 mm	1.5° Flex
Deviation	0.5° Var	+1.0 mm	1.5° Flex

For the sake of understanding and building an algorithm for FFD correction, we have divided them as under:

- <10-degree FFD.
- 10- to 20-degree FFD.
- 20- to 30-degree FFD.
- 30- to 40-degree FFD.
- >50-degree FFD.

<10-degree FFD

- Full-length radiographs of the lower limb with anteroposterior and lateral views of the right knee (**Fig. 5.2**).
- The X-ray revealed tricompartmental arthritis with neutral coronal alignment.
- Lateral view of the patient suggestive of FFD at the knee joint.

- Navigation revealed neutral coronal alignment of the limb with 10-degree flexion deformity in the sagittal plane (**Fig. 5.3**).
- +1 mm extra distal femoral cut was taken to increase the extension space (**Fig. 5.4**).
- An accurate distal femoral cut is the key operative step in increasing the extension space to achieve neutral alignment with final components (**Fig. 5.5**).
- Navigation values show the verification of the proximal tibial cut (**Fig. 5.6**).
- The final kinematic graph revealed complete correction of the deformity both in sagittal and coronal planes (**Fig. 5.7**).
- The knee was kept in residual flexion of 3 degrees, which usually stretches out to neutral on weight-bearing.

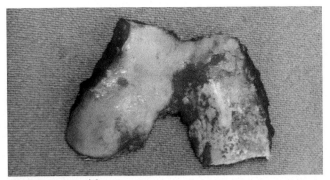

Fig. 5.5   Distal femur cut.

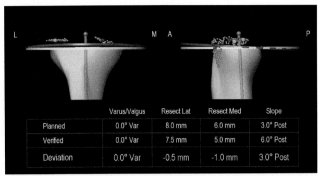

Fig. 5.6   Proximal tibia cut verification

	Varus/Valgus	Resect Lat	Resect Med	Slope
Planned	0.0° Var	8.0 mm	6.0 mm	3.0° Post
Verified	0.0° Var	7.5 mm	5.0 mm	6.0° Post
Deviation	0.0° Var	-0.5 mm	-1.0 mm	3.0° Post

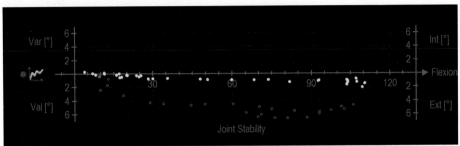

Fig. 5.7   Final limb alignment and kinematics.

- Postoperative anteroposterior and lateral views of the knee revealed well-implanted femoral and tibial components (**Fig. 5.8**).

Pearls

- Not all FFDs require an additional distal femur cut for correction. Repeated evaluation of the flexion and extension gaps is advised after the execution of each surgical step.
- For every 10 degree of FFD, an extra millimeter of distal femoral cut may be required to correct the FFD, provided there are no large posterior osteophytes.
- If FFD is associated with large posterior osteophytes then their removal is likely to correct FFD.

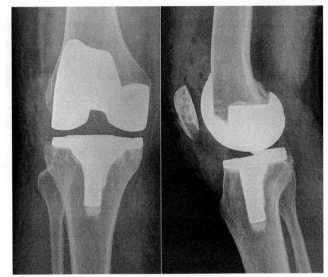

Fig. 5.8   Postoperative radiographs.

10- to 20-degree FFD

- Preoperative knee X-rays elicit osteoarthritis, negligible posterior osteophytes, suggesting a tight posterior capsule as a potential cause for FFD (**Fig. 5.9**).
- Clinical evaluation showing FFD in standing and supine position (**Fig. 5.10**).
- The preoperative kinematic analysis demonstrates severe flexion deformity of 17.5 degrees with minimal correctable varus of 4 degrees (**Fig. 5.11**).
- Distal femoral cut can be accurately titrated based on extent of fixed flexion deformity (**Fig. 5.12**).
- An additional 1 to 2 mm of the distal femoral cut was required for this particular flexion deformity in addition to release of the posterior capsule.
- The major advantage of navigation is to precisely quantify the sagittal plane deformity and plan the DFC accordingly.

- Verification of the proximal tibia cut was performed (**Fig. 5.13**).
- In cases with flexion deformity, the extension gap is tighter than the flexion gap.
- This laxity in the flexion gap is managed by either upsizing the femoral component, decreasing the tibial slope or both.
- The ability to accurately adjust the tibial slope and analyze its effects on balancing the knee is yet another advantage of computer navigation.

Pearls

In cases with FFD, the posterior slope can be kept in between 1 and 3 degrees to snug the flexion space and aid gap balancing.

- Anterior slope should be strictly avoided.
- More than 3 degrees of posterior slope increases flexion gap causing gap imbalance (**Fig. 5.14**).

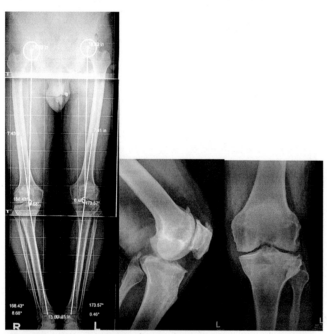

Fig. 5.9 Preoperative radiographs.

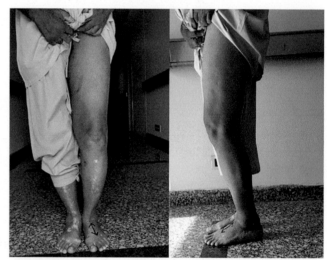

Fig. 5.10 Clinical image of the patient.

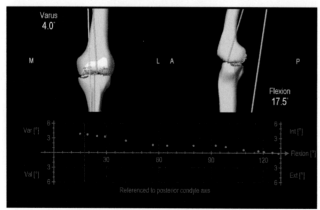

Fig. 5.11 Initial limb alignment and kinematics.

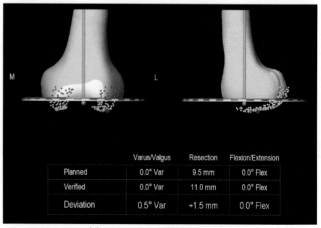

	Varus/Valgus	Resection	Flexion/Extension
Planned	0.0° Var	9.5 mm	0.0° Flex
Verified	0.0° Var	11.0 mm	0.0° Flex
Deviation	0.5° Var	+1.5 mm	0.0° Flex

Fig. 5.12 Distal femur cut verification.

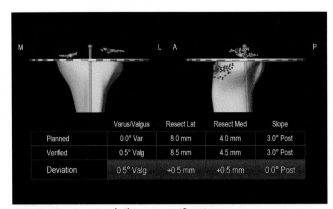

Fig. 5.13 Proximal tibia cut verification.

- Removal of posterior tibial osteophytes relives capsular tension and increases extension gap (**Fig. 5.15**).
- Final kinematics and limb alignment analysis revealed the correction of flexion deformity (**Fig. 5.16**).

- Postoperative anteroposterior and lateral radiographs of the knee revealed the appropriate placement of components (**Fig. 5.17**).

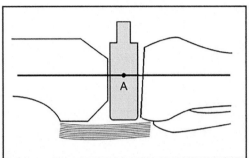
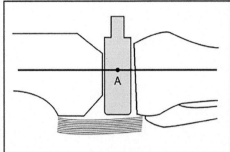

Fig. 5.14 Effect of tibial slope on extension gap.

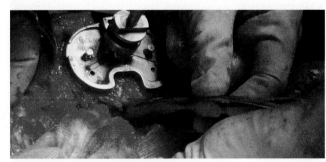

Fig. 5.15 Posterior osteophytes removal

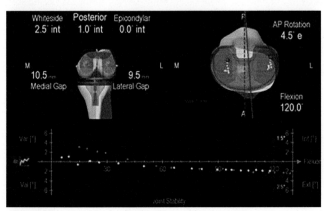

Fig. 5.16 Final limb alignment and kinematics.

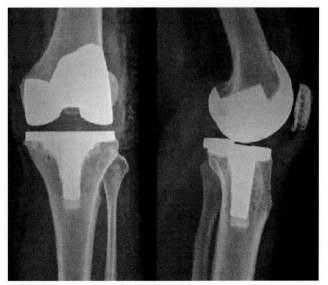

Fig. 5.17 Postoperative radiographs.

20- to 30-degree FFD

- Tricompartmental arthritis with posterior osteophytes can be seen in preoperative radiographs (**Fig. 5.18**).
- Clinical examination revealed 25 degrees of FFD, with further flexion up to 105 degrees (**Fig. 5.19**).
- Preoperative kinematics analysis demonstrated a limited range of movement with flexion deformity (**Fig. 5.20**).
- A normal distal femoral resection was performed, as the knee had large posterior osteophytes and was subluxed in this case (**Fig. 5.21**).

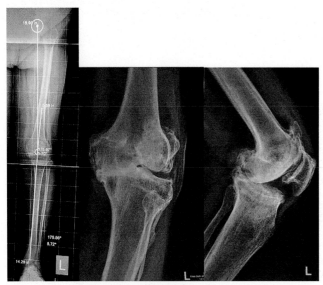

Fig. 5.18 Preoperative radiographs

Neurovascular status should always be checked pre- and postoperatively after correction of severe FFD.

- A proximal tibial cut with 1- to 3-degree posterior slope to balance the flexion gap (**Fig. 5.22**).

Pitfalls

- Posterior osteophytes limit both extension and flexion.
- Tenting and scarring of the posterior capsule causes decreased extension while impingement of the osteophytes with the femoral condyles causes decreased ROM.
- Long-standing FFD may lead to hamstring contracture.

- Intraoperative image showing the removal of the posterior osteophytes and elevation of capsule from posterior aspect of tibia (**Fig. 5.23**).
- The posterior capsule was also lifted with cautery and osteotome to gain extension.
- No additional distal femur cut was required in this case as FFD was associated with the presence of posterior osteophytes and adhesions of the posterior capsule.
- Complete correction of the sagittal and coronal plane deformity seen in postoperative kinematics (**Fig. 5.24**).
- Postoperative radiographs show well-aligned femoral and tibial components (**Fig. 5.25**).

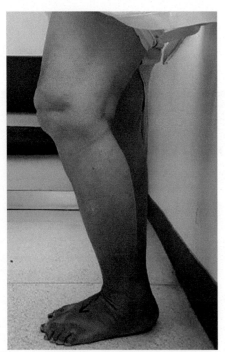

Fig. 5.19 Clinical image of the patient showing severe fixed flexion deformity (FFD).

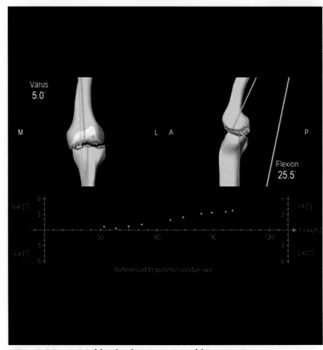

Fig. 5.20 Initial limb alignment and kinematics.

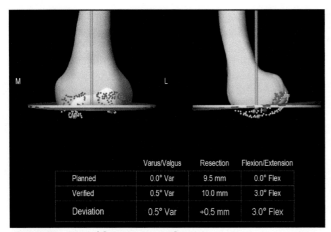

	Varus/Valgus	Resection	Flexion/Extension
Planned	0.0° Var	9.5 mm	0.0° Flex
Verified	0.5° Var	10.0 mm	3.0° Flex
Deviation	0.5° Var	+0.5 mm	3.0° Flex

Fig. 5.21   Distal femur cut verification.

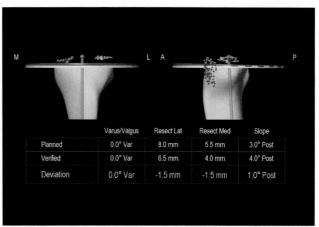

	Varus/Valgus	Resect Lat	Resect Med	Slope
Planned	0.0° Var	8.0 mm	5.5 mm	3.0° Post
Verified	0.0° Var	6.5 mm	4.0 mm	4.0° Post
Deviation	0.0° Var	-1.5 mm	-1.5 mm	1.0° Post

Fig. 5.22   Proximal tibia cut verification.

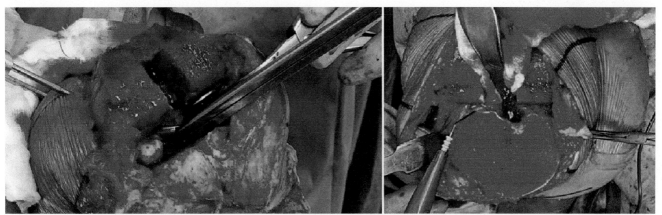

Fig. 5.23   Posterior osteophytes removal and elevation of capsule from posterior aspect of tibia.

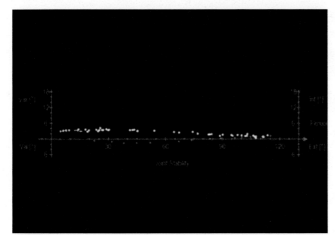

Fig. 5.24   Postoperative limb alignment and kinematics.

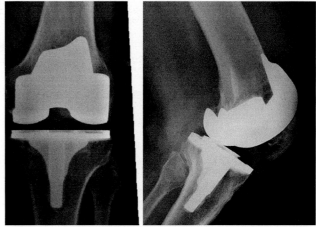

Fig. 5.25   Postoperative radiographs.

30- to 40-degree FFD

- The preoperative radiographs and clinical images revealed tricompartmental arthritis of bilateral knee joints with the presence of posterior and suprapatellar osteophytes resulting in significant FFD (**Fig. 5.26** to **Fig. 5.29**).
- 38-degree FFD with negligible varus seen in preoperative kinematics graph.
- The intercondylar osteophytes cause bony impingement and result in decreased extension.
- The osteophytes should be removed before assessing the residual FFD.
- An additional distal femur resection of +3.5 mm was performed to increase the extension gap (**Fig. 5.30**).

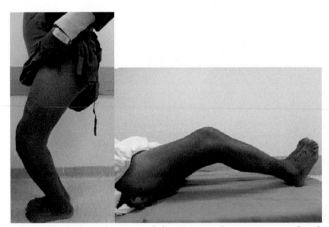

Fig. 5.26 Clinical image of the patient showing severe fixed flexion deformity (FFD).

- Distal femur cut of more than 13 to 14 mm is not recommended, as it may damage the collateral ligaments attachments.
- Excess distal femur cut may also significantly alter the joint line, resulting in disturbed knee kinematics.
- An intraoperative picture showing the release of the posteromedial capsule, correcting the associated deformity (**Fig. 5.31**).
- An additional proximal tibial resection with a 1- to 3-degree posterior slope helped balance the loose flexion gap (**Fig. 5.32**).
- Navigation accurately predicted the relationship of the bony cut with the defect present on the medial tibial condyle.

Pearls

If there is severe FFD without associated coronal plane deformity, then a balanced approach of resecting extra bone on both distal femur and tibia should be employed. This will keep joint line intact ensuring patellar tracking and balanced knee.

Patella Baja

- Patella baja, if associated with FFD, makes the deformity correction more challenging.
- There is an increased risk of patellar impingement on the insert along with a decreased range of motion of the knee.
- Excessive distal femur cut along with a conservative tibial cut would worsen the patella baja.

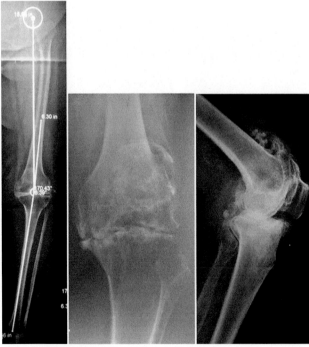

Fig. 5.27 Preoperative radiographs of left knee.

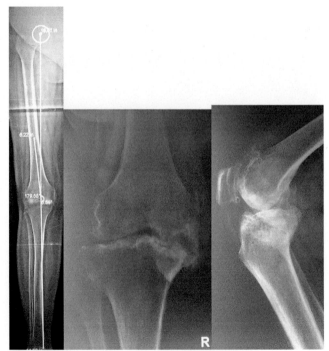

Fig. 5.28 Preoperative radiographs of right knee.

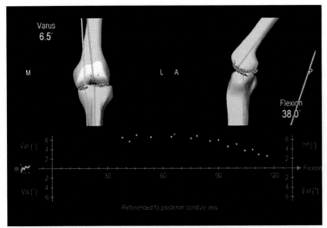

Fig. 5.29 Initial limb alignment and kinematics.

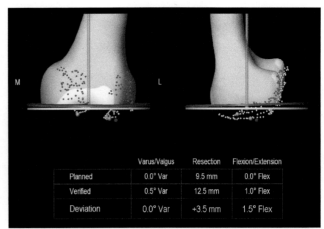

	Varus/Valgus	Resection	Flexion/Extension
Planned	0.0° Var	9.5 mm	0.0° Flex
Verified	0.5° Var	12.5 mm	1.0° Flex
Deviation	0.0° Var	+3.5 mm	1.5° Flex

Fig. 5.30 Distal femur cut and verification.

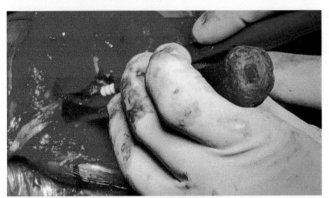

Fig. 5.31 Posteromedial capsule elevation.

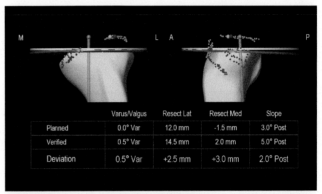

	Varus/Valgus	Resect Lat	Resect Med	Slope
Planned	0.0° Var	12.0 mm	-1.5 mm	3.0° Post
Verified	0.5° Var	14.5 mm	2.0 mm	5.0° Post
Deviation	0.5° Var	+2.5 mm	+3.0 mm	2.0° Post

Fig. 5.32 Proximal tibial cut verification.

- Carefully analyze the preoperative radiographs for patella baja.
- An +1 to + 3 mm extra distal femur cut with an increased tibial cut and decreased posterior slope is advised.
- While preparing the patella, it is advisable to place the patellar button superiorly to avoid impingement of the patella on the poly (**Fig. 5.33**).
- A high-flexion insert with a smooth anterior chamfer is recommended to prevent patellar impingement on poly.
- The postoperative kinematic graph revealed the complete correction of the sagittal and coronal plane deformities (yellow dots) (**Fig. 5.34**).
- Postoperative radiographs demonstrated well-aligned prosthetic components (**Fig. 5.35**).
- Complete correction of sagittal and coronal plane deformity seen in postoperative clinical image. (**Fig. 5.36**).

- A short knee brace should be recommended postoperatively, especially at night.
- Avoid usage of continuous passive motion (CPM), as it keeps the knee in flexion.

Pearls

- If severe FFD is present bilaterally, the authors recommend correcting both the knees either simultaneously or within a short time frame.
- There are higher chances of recurrence of a flexion deformity.
- Strict follow-up is necessary in initial period to identify recurrence of deformity.
- Extended physiotherapy can be recommended to the patients showing poor compliance.

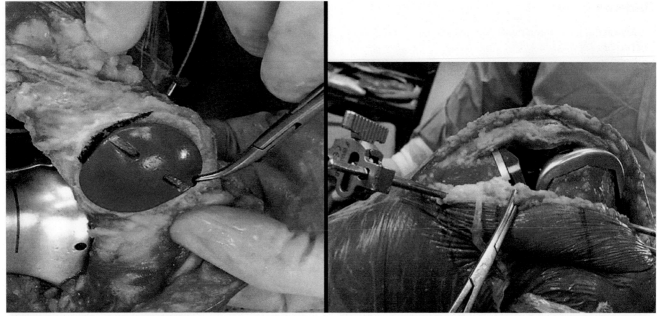

Fig. 5.33 Patellar baja correction.

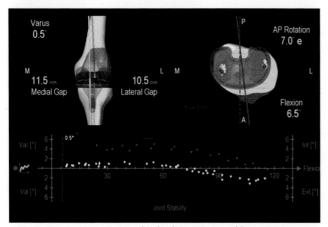

Fig. 5.34 Postoperative limb alignment and kinematics.

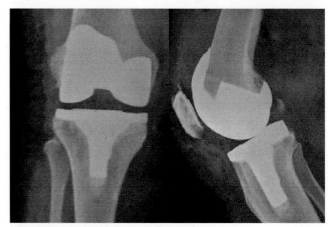

Fig. 5.35 Postoperative radiographs.

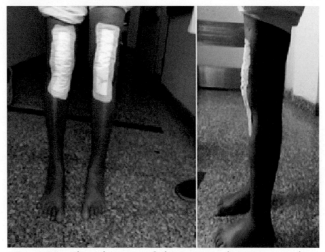

Fig. 5.36 Clinical image of the patient showing complete correction of sagittal deformity.

50-degree FFD

- Advanced, tricompartment osteoarthritis seen in preoperative radiographs (**Fig. 5.37** and **Fig. 5.38**).
- Preoperative navigation kinematics show 51 degrees of FFD with restricted range of movement (**Fig. 5.39**).
- Navigation didn't reveal any associated coronal plane deformity as the knee was in significant flexion.
- A 4 to 5 mm of extra distal femoral resection was performed to achieve an optimum extension gap (**Fig. 5.40**).
- Extra caution is advocated to prevent iatrogenic damage to the collateral ligaments.

- An extra distal femur cut of +4 to +5 can damage the collateral ligaments. Angel wing should be passed to assess the exit path of the saw before proceeding for a large distal femur cut (**Fig. 5.41**).
- An additional proximal tibial cut was taken with a decreased posterior slope to achieve the gap balance (**Fig. 5.42**).
- Removal of posterior osteophytes increases extension gap (**Fig. 5.43**).
- Posteromedial capsule was released with the help of bent cautery tip to relieve soft tissue tension (**Fig. 5.44**)

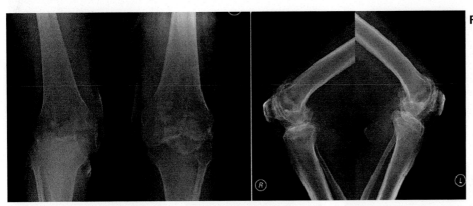

Fig. 5.37 Preoperative radiographs.

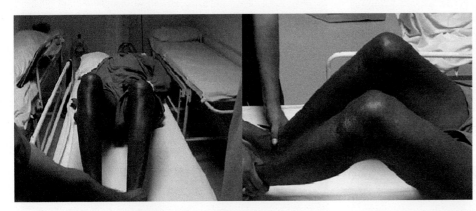

Fig. 5.38 Clinical image of the patient.

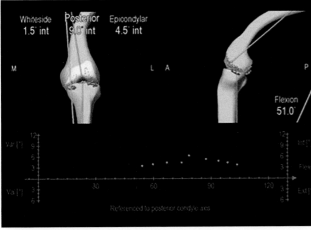

Fig. 5.39 Preoperative limb alignment and kinematics.

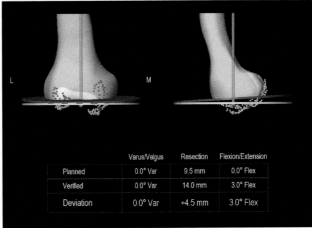

Fig. 5.40 Distal femur cut and verification.

	Varus/Valgus	Resection	Flexion/Extension
Planned	0.0° Var	9.5 mm	0.0° Flex
Verified	0.0° Var	14.0 mm	3.0° Flex
Deviation	0.0° Var	+4.5 mm	3.0° Flex

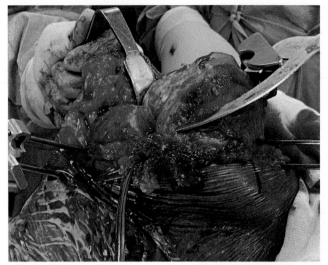

Fig. 5.41 Distal femur cut should not violate collateral ligament (MCL).

- The postoperative navigation kinematics graph demonstrated a significantly increased range of motion with correction of the deformity (**Fig. 5.45**).
- For gradual correction of the residual 10 degree of FFD, a knee brace and passive stretching of the knee was advised postoperatively.
- Usually, the residual flexion deformities improve with physiotherapy and posterior capsular stretching on weight-bearing.

Pearls

- Percutaneous tenotomy of hamstrings may be needed in severe resistant cases of FFD where all bony cuts and soft tissue releases do not correct FFD fully.
- Keep a roll or a bolster under the ankle to keep the knee in extension.

- Postoperative radiographs demonstrated well-aligned knee components (**Fig. 5.46**).

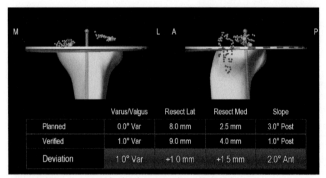

	Varus/Valgus	Resect Lat	Resect Med	Slope
Planned	0.0° Var	8.0 mm	2.5 mm	3.0° Post
Verified	1.0° Var	9.0 mm	4.0 mm	1.0° Post
Deviation	1.0° Var	+1.0 mm	+1.5 mm	2.0° Ant

Fig. 5.42 Proximal tibial cut and verification.

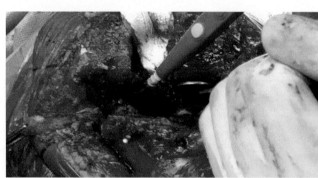

Fig. 5.44 Posteromedial capsule elevation.

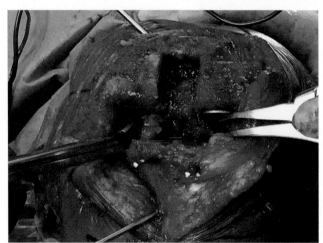

Fig. 5.43 Posterior osteophytes removal.

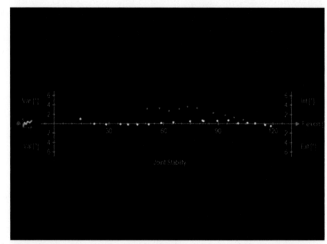

Fig. 5.45 Postoperative limb alignment and kinematics.

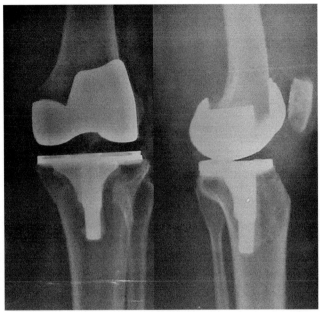

Fig. 5.46 Postoperative radiographs.

Points to Remember

For severe FFD cases, the decision to correct the deformity fully depends on the etiology of the deformity:

- FFD due to an inflammatory origin such as rheumatoid arthritis can be left in 5- to 10-degree flexion as it stretches out with time and weight-bearing.
- FFD of traumatic origin or osteoarthritis needs complete correction intraoperatively, as such deformities are chronic and have secondary hamstring contracture, which forces the knee to go in flexion postoperatively.
- Adequate removal of the posterior osteophytes and posterior capsular release can significantly aid in the correction of FFD.
- Patients in FFD preoperatively have a greater tendency to keep their knees in flexion postoperatively.
- Knee extension immobilizers, bolster under the ankle, or short-term splinting can be advised to prevent recurrence of the deformity in the postoperative period.

References

1. Abdelaal AHK, Yamamoto N, Hayashi K, et al. Radiological assessment of the femoral bowing in Japanese population. SICOT J 2016;2:2

2. Aderinto J, Brenkel IJ, Chan P. Natural history of fixed flexion deformity following knee replacement. J Bone Joint Surg Br 2005;87:934–936

3. Su EP. Fixed flexion deformity and total knee arthroplasty. J Bone Joint Surg Br 2012; 94(11, Suppl A):112–115

4. Lam LO, Swift S, Shakespeare D. Fixed flexion deformity and flexion after knee arthroplasty. What happens in the first 12 months after surgery and can a poor outcome be predicted? Knee 2003;10(2):181–185

5. Tew M, Forster IW. Effect of knee replacement on flexion deformity. J Bone Joint Surg Br 1987;69(3):395–399

6. Bhave A, Mont M, Tennis S, Nickey M, Starr R, Etienne G. Functional problems and treatment solutions after total hip and knee joint arthroplasty. J Bone Joint Surg Am 2005;87(Suppl 2):9–21

7. McPherson EJ, Cushner FD, Schiff CF, Friedman RJ. Natural history of uncorrected flexion contractures following total knee arthroplasty. J Arthroplasty 1994;9(5):499–502

8. Sultan PG, Most E, Schule S, Li G, Rubash HE. Optimizing flexion after total knee arthroplasty: advances in prosthetic design. Clin Orthop Relat Res. 2003;(416):167–173

9. Okazaki K, Tashiro Y, Mizu-uchi H, Hamai S, Doi T, Iwamoto Y. Influence of the posterior tibial slope on the flexion gap in total knee arthroplasty. Knee 2014;21(4):806–809

Computer-Navigated TKR for Recurvatum Deformity

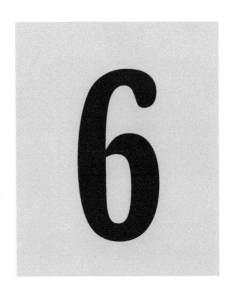

Anoop Jhurani and Piyush Agarwal

Introduction

- A normal knee may have recurvatum up to 3 degrees. A knee with more than 3-degree hyperextension can be considered a recurvatum deformity.
- Recurvatum deformity is difficult to diagnose with the patient lying supine. It unmasks itself in stance phase of gait or after anesthesia. Thus, every patient undergoing knee replacement should be examined carefully while walking and after spinal anesthesia.
- The reported incidence of this deformity varies from 1 to 10% depending upon the patient's ethnicity, race, and surgical technique used.[1]
- With the advent of computer navigation, recurvatum deformities are being accurately diagnosed and precisely quantified, leading to increase in reported incidence.
- Conventional TKA in patients with recurvatum may result in recurrence and suboptimal outcomes because of failure to recognize this subtle deformity.

Causes of Recurvatum Deformity in Knees[2]

- Anterior femoral or tibial bone loss.
- Inflammatory disorders like rheumatoid arthritis.
- Post–high tibial osteotomy (HTO).
- Posterior capsular or ligamentous laxity.
- Neuromuscular disorders like poliomyelitis.
- Neuropathic knee.

Advantages of Using Computer Navigation for Recurvatum Knees

- Accurate assessment and precise quantification of the recurvatum deformity preoperatively.
- Assistance in planning the bony cuts intraoperatively, to rectify the deformity and achieve a well-balanced, stable knee.
- It further aids in balancing the knee without additional need for constrained implants or thicker inserts.
- The extent of recurvatum deformity along with any associated coronal plane deformity is taken into account to modify the bony cuts, in order to achieve a well-balanced knee.

Recommended Surgical Steps to Correct Hyperextension Deformity[3–6]

- Reduced bony resection of distal femur and tibia.
- Undersizing the femoral component and minimal soft tissue release.
- Tightening the extension gap using thicker inserts.
- Using distal femoral augments.
- Constrained or hinged knee in neuropathic knees.
- Proximal and posterior transfer of the collateral ligaments.
- In this chapter, the principles and an algorithm for the correction of a recurvatum deformity is outlined.

Biomechanics of Recurvatum Deformity

- The ground reaction forces lie slightly anterior to the center of gravity of knee on weight bearing which helps in maintaining fine balance between hamstrings and quadriceps.
- It allows knee to get locked in extension during stance phase.
- In knees with recurvatum, there is forward leaning of the trunk on weight-bearing which causes the resultant ground reaction forces to shift anterior to the knee.

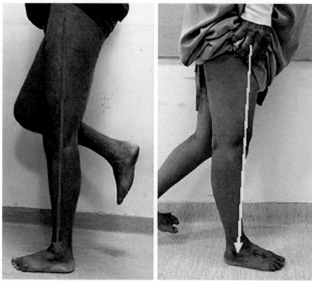

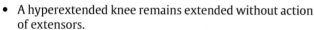

Fig. 6.1 Resultant ground reaction forces in normal knee and knee with recurvatum deformity.

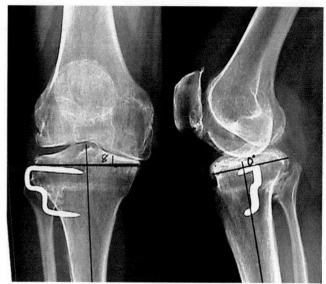

Fig. 6.2 Preoperative anteroposterior (AP) and lateral view of knee.

- A hyperextended knee remains extended without action of extensors.
- It leads to further stretching of the posterior capsule of the knee.
- This causes decreased walking distance, instability, and difficulty in balancing.
- Resultant ground reaction force in normal knee and in knee with recurvatum (**Fig. 6.1**).

Principles

- A reduction in the extent of distal femoral cut with or without a reduction in proximal tibial cut may be required for a balanced knee in whole arc of motion (Whiteside and Milhalko principle).[6]
- Theoretically, this approach may lead to a change in the joint line which may affect the joint biomechanics resulting in suboptimal clinical outcomes.[6]

- However, our data suggests that most recurvatum knees are lax globally with an equally loose flexion space, thus requiring a conservative tibial cut.[7]
- For ease of understanding the behavior and management of recurvatum knees we have divided them in following four categories:
  - <5-degree recurvatum.
  - 5- to 10-degree recurvatum.
  - 10- to 15-degree recurvatum.
  - 15-degree recurvatum.

<5-degree Recurvatum

- Conventional lateral closing wedge osteotomy was done for this patient 10 years back.

- There is minimal coronal plane deformity with valgus joint line and staple in situ.
- Reversal of tibial slope can be seen in lateral view (**Fig. 6.2**).
- Post-HTO cases generally present with recurvatum deformity because of loss of anterior tibial bone and reversal of tibial slope.[8]
- The navigation graph showed minimal deformity in coronal plane with 5-degree recurvatum (**Fig. 6.3**).
- A reduction of 0.5 to 1 mm of the distal femur cut is sufficient to achieve balanced gap in extension (**Fig. 6.4**).
- Such precision in planning the bony cuts can be achieved with the help of computer navigation.
- Measured resection of the proximal tibial cut equalized the flexion and extension gaps (**Fig. 6.5**).
- The postoperative kinematics graph revealed a balanced flexion and extension gap, with correction of the preoperative deformity (**Fig. 6.6**).
- The anteroposterior and lateral radiographs of the patient elicit well-fixed and well-aligned prosthetic components (**Fig. 6.7**).

Pearls

- The patients starting with a recurvatum deformity are prone to recurrence of the hyperextension postoperatively.
- This is because of the tendency of the posterior capsule to stretch on weight-bearing.
- Thus, it is advisable to keep such knees in 5- to 7-degree of flexion postoperatively.

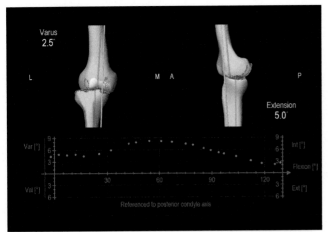

Fig. 6.3 Preoperative limb alignment and kinematics.

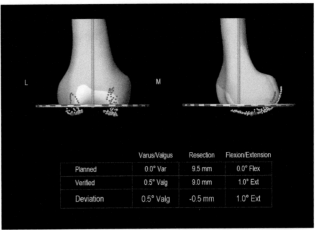

Fig. 6.4 Distal femoral cut verification.

	Varus/Valgus	Resection	Flexion/Extension
Planned	0.0° Var	9.5 mm	0.0° Flex
Verified	0.5° Valg	9.0 mm	1.0° Ext
Deviation	0.5° Valg	-0.5 mm	1.0° Ext

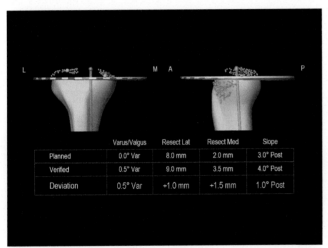

Fig. 6.5 Tibial resection verification.

	Varus/Valgus	Resect Lat	Resect Med	Slope
Planned	0.0° Var	8.0 mm	2.0 mm	3.0° Post
Verified	0.5° Var	9.0 mm	3.5 mm	4.0° Post
Deviation	0.5° Var	+1.0 mm	+1.5 mm	1.0° Post

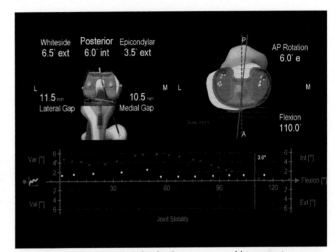

Fig. 6.6 Postoperative limb alignment and kinematics.

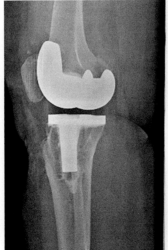

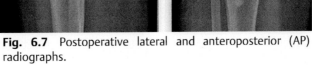

Fig. 6.7 Postoperative lateral and anteroposterior (AP) radiographs.

5- to 10-degree Recurvatum

- The preoperative radiographs show mild varus deformity with bone on bone arthritis in the medial compartment and opening up of the lateral compartment (**Fig. 6.8**).
- Recurvatum deformity can be seen in preoperative clinical picture.
- The preoperative kinematic analysis demonstrated increased deformity in the sagittal plane than in the coronal plane (**Fig. 6.9**).

Pearls

- A patient with a recurvatum deformity complains of difficulty in walking than pain in the knee joint.
- Such patients usually have a feeling of the knee giving away or buckling.

- An underresection of -1.5 mm of the distal femur was done to balance the loose extension gap (**Fig. 6.10**).
- Recurvatum deformities usually exhibit an equally lax flexion gap (**Fig. 6.11**).
- Hence, underresection of the tibia was done to balance the knee with minimal insert thickness (9 mm).
- The postoperative kinematic alignment demonstrated the correction of deformity with residual 3- to 5-degree flexion postoperatively (**Fig. 6.12**).
- Well-aligned components in postoperative anteroposterior and lateral views (**Fig. 6.13**).
- A clinical picture depicting complete correction of the recurvatum deformity.

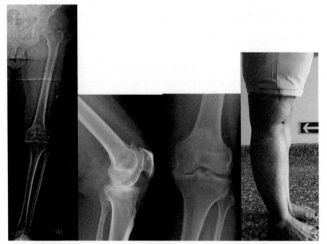

Fig. 6.8 Preoperative radiographs and lateral view of patient's knee.

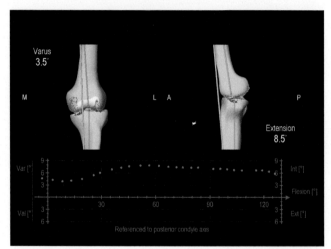

Fig. 6.9 Preoperative limb alignment and kinematics.

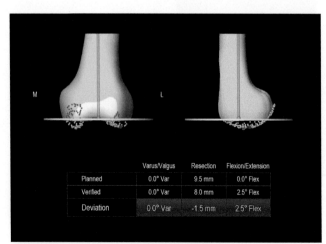

	Varus/Valgus	Resection	Flexion/Extension
Planned	0.0° Var	9.5 mm	0.0° Flex
Verified	0.0° Var	8.0 mm	2.5° Flex
Deviation	0.0° Var	-1.5 mm	2.5° Flex

Fig. 6.10 Distal femur cut verification.

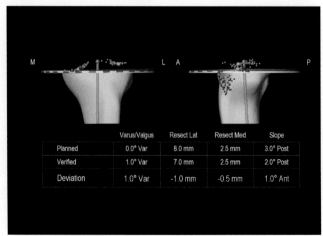

	Varus/Valgus	Resect Lat	Resect Med	Slope
Planned	0.0° Var	8.0 mm	2.5 mm	3.0° Post
Verified	1.0° Var	7.0 mm	2.5 mm	2.0° Post
Deviation	1.0° Var	-1.0 mm	-0.5 mm	1.0° Ant

Fig. 6.11 Tibial resection verification.

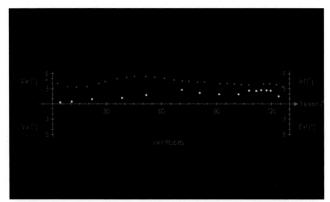

Fig. 6.12 Postoperative limb alignment and kinematics.

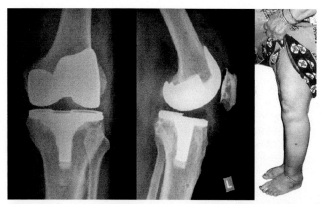

Fig. 6.13 Postoperative anteroposterior (AP) and lateral radiographs with sagittal limb alignment at 2-year follow-up.

10- to 15-degree Recurvatum

- Posttraumatic arthritis with gross destruction of the articular surface of the knee with patella alta can be seen in preoperative radiographs (**Fig. 6.14**).
- An intraoperative clinical picture depicting recurvatum deformity at the knee (**Fig. 6.15**).
- Navigation accurately showing distorted proximal tibial anatomy (**Fig. 6.16**).
- There was femoral subluxation resulting in 15-degree recurvatum deformity.
- As the knee was subluxed with 15 degree of hyperextension, its coronal alignment showed 1.5-degree varus with overall valgus alignment throughout ROM.

Pitfalls

- In subluxed knee with global instability, coronal alignment may change depending on the way surgeon holds the knee in extension.
- Knee should be kept in neutral position without varus or valgus stress while registering deformity.

- To compensate for the loose extension gap, underresection of the distal femur by -2 mm was performed (**Fig. 6.17**).

- However, one has to exert caution as excessive reduction of the distal femoral cut can potentially hamper the patellar tracking.
- Minimal distal femur cut of 6 mm (**Fig. 6.18**).
- External rotation was kept at 5 degrees to compensate for lateral opening (**Fig. 6.19**).
- It could be increased to compensate for lateral opening.
- Navigation accurately depicted the altered posterior slope and surface morphology of proximal tibia (**Fig. 6.20**).
- The residual medial tibial condyle defect could be seen after the planned tibial cut.
- The navigation values showed the orientation of the tibial cut in all the three planes (thickness, posterior slope, varus/valgus angulation) (**Fig. 6.21**).
- Minimal tibial cut of 5 mm to compensate for loose extension and flexion space (**Fig. 6.22**).
- A complete correction of the preoperative deformity can be seen in postoperative kinematic graph (**Fig. 6.23**).
- The knee was left in 5 to 7 degrees of residual flexion to prevent any reoccurrence of recurvatum deformity on weight bearing.
- The tibial baseplate was augmented by a tibial extension rod for load sharing in osteoporotic bone (**Fig. 6.24**).
- Two bone screws and cement were also used to manage the bone defect on the medial tibial condyle.

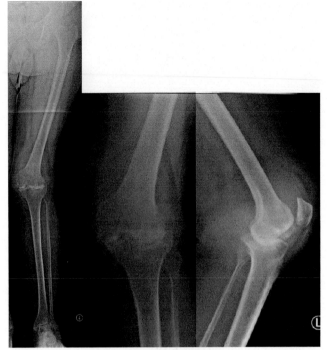

Fig. 6.14 Preoperative radiographs.

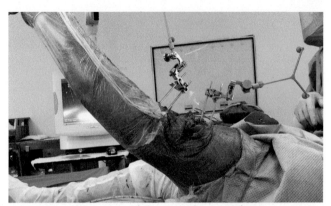

Fig. 6.15 Recurvatum deformity after anesthesia.

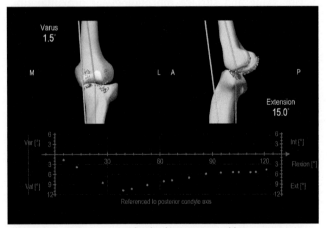

Fig. 6.16 Preoperative limb alignment and kinematics.

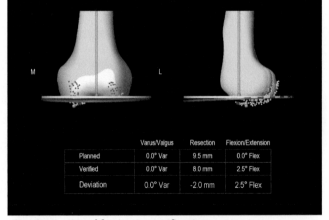

	Varus/Valgus	Resection	Flexion/Extension
Planned	0.0° Var	9.5 mm	0.0° Flex
Verified	0.0° Var	8.0 mm	2.5° Flex
Deviation	0.0° Var	-2.0 mm	2.5° Flex

Fig. 6.17 Distal femur cut verification.

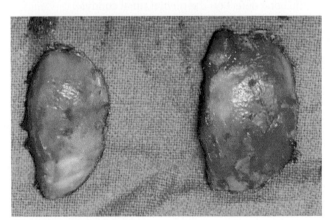

Fig. 6.18 Distal femur cut.

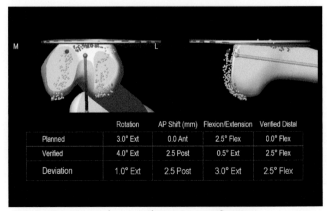

	Rotation	AP Shift (mm)	Flexion/Extension	Verified Distal
Planned	3.0° Ext	0.0 Ant	2.5° Flex	0.0° Flex
Verified	4.0° Ext	2.5 Post	0.5° Ext	2.5° Flex
Deviation	1.0° Ext	2.5 Post	3.0° Ext	2.5° Flex

Fig. 6.19 Femoral external rotation verification.

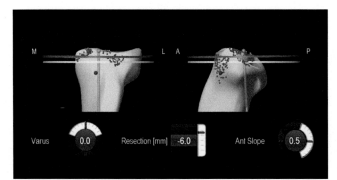

Fig. 6.20 Proximal tibia 3D model.

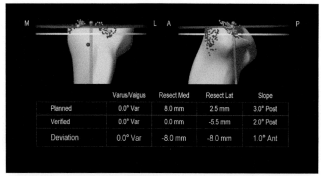

Fig. 6.21 Tibial cut verification.

	Varus/Valgus	Resect Med	Resect Lat	Slope
Planned	0.0° Var	8.0 mm	2.5 mm	3.0° Post
Verified	0.0° Var	0.0 mm	-5.5 mm	2.0° Post
Deviation	0.0° Var	-8.0 mm	-8.0 mm	1.0° Ant

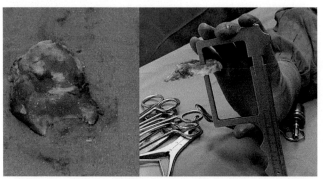

Fig. 6.22 Proximal tibia cut.

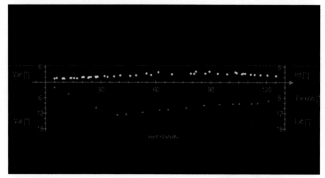

Fig. 6.23 Postoperative limb alignment and kinematics.

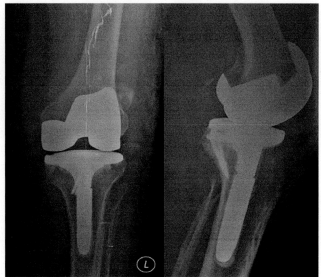

Fig. 6.24 Postoperative anteroposterior (AP) and lateral radiographs.

>15-degree Recurvatum

- This is the case of a 75-year-old female having history of spinal surgery with clinical features of neuropathic joint.
- Subluxation of the tibiofemoral joint and tricompartmental arthritis seen on preoperative radiographs (**Fig. 6.25**).
- On examination, the patient had a subluxed knee with mediolateral instability.
- The patient's ROM was 15 degrees of recurvatum, flexion up to 90 degrees with 25 degrees of varus.
- This case had a biplanar deformity with predominant varus deformity associated with severe recurvatum, making it unstable globally.
- It required higher constraint prosthesis to maintain the stability in the sagittal and coronal planes.
- This case is an example where careful clinical evaluation of the patient and the radiographs before surgery helps in determining the level of constraint to be used intraoperatively.
- The preoperative kinematics demonstrated a severe varus-recurvatum deformity. Although this was a biplanar deformity, this case was included here to elicit the management of knees with a lax posterior capsule and concomitant ligamentous instability (**Fig. 6.26**).
- The soft tissue correction of the varus deformity can increase the recurvatum deformity, due to the relaxation of the posteromedial capsule.
- As a consequence of the gross instability, a rotating hinge knee was planned in this case.
- A minimal distal femoral resection was performed to help reduce the extension gap (**Fig. 6.27**).
- A conservative proximal tibial resection was performed to balance the knee with the requirement of a minimal thickness insert (**Fig. 6.28**).
- Complete correction of the deformity in both the planes, with balanced knee can be seen in postoperative kinematics (**Fig. 6.29**).
- The postoperative radiographs show the correction of deformity with a rotating hinge knee system which was used to prevent recurrence of recurvatum deformity in neuropathic joint (**Fig. 6.30**).

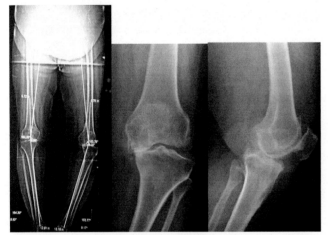

Fig. 6.25 Preoperative radiographs.

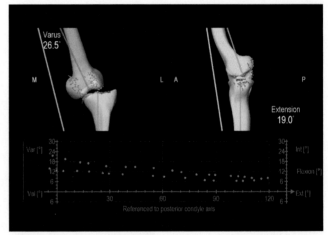

Fig. 6.26 Preoperative limb alignment and kinematics.

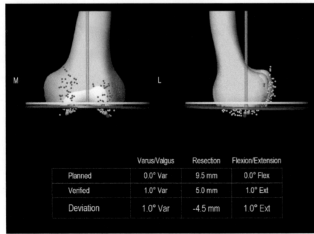

	Varus/Valgus	Resection	Flexion/Extension
Planned	0.0° Var	9.5 mm	0.0° Flex
Verified	1.0° Var	5.0 mm	1.0° Ext
Deviation	1.0° Var	-4.5 mm	1.0° Ext

Fig. 6.27 Distal femur cut verification.

	Varus/Valgus	Resect Lat	Resect Med	Slope
Planned	0.0° Var	8.0 mm	3.5 mm	3.0° Post
Verified	0.0° Var	5.0 mm	0.5 mm	2.5° Post
Deviation	0.0° Var	-3.0 mm	-3.0 mm	0.5° Ant

Fig. 6.28 Tibial cut verification.

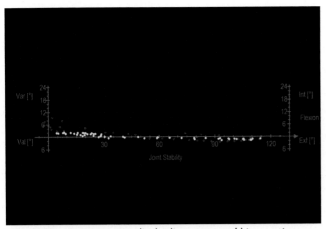

Fig. 6.29 Postoperative limb alignment and kinematics.

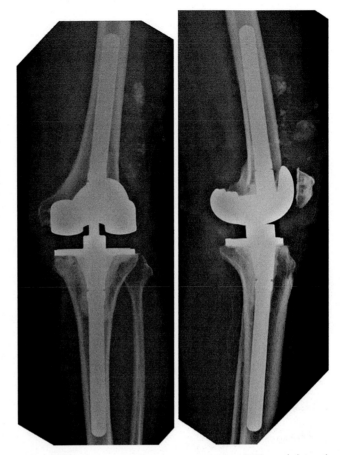

Fig. 6.30 Postoperative anteroposterior (AP) and lateral radiographs.

Pitfalls

- Computer navigation has the limitation of not predicting or recommending the extent of bony resection required, relying on the operating surgeon's decision based on the type and severity of deformity present in each case.
- This limitation is overcome by robotic assisted surgery, which not only predicts soft tissue behavior but also guides the surgeon in intraoperative decision making.

Points to Remember

- The authors advise to leave the recurvatum knees in 5 to 7 degrees of flexion postoperatively to prevent recurrence of recurvatum on weight-bearing due to stretching of posterior capsule.
- However, a knee kept in >10 degrees of fixed flexion postoperatively would result in compromised clinical outcomes, due to impaired quadriceps function.[9]
- Leaving a recurvatum knee in neutral sagittal or slight recurvatum alignment postoperatively may lead to a recurrence of deformity on follow-up, especially in cases with inflammatory arthritis or neuropathic knees.[10]
- This would lead to difficulty in walking postoperatively and an early box-cam failure.[10]

References

1. Siddiqui MM, Yeo SJ, Sivaiah P, Chia SL, Chin PL, Lo NN. Function and quality of life in patients with recurvatum deformity after primary total knee arthroplasty: a review of our joint registry. J Arthroplasty 2012;27(6):1106–1110

2. Mullaji A, Lingaraju AP, Shetty GM. Computer-assisted total knee replacement in patients with arthritis and a recurvatum deformity. J Bone Joint Surg Br 2012;94(5):642–647

3. Meding JB, Keating EM, Ritter MA, Faris PM, Berend ME. Genu recurvatum in total knee replacement. Clin Orthop Relat Res 2003; (416):64–67

4. Parratte S, Pagnano MW. Instability after total knee arthroplasty. J Bone Joint Surg Am 2008;90(1):184–194

5. Insall JN. Surgical techniques and instrumentation in total knee arthroplasty. In: Insall JN, Windsor RE, Scott WN, Kelly MA, Aglietti P, eds. Surgery of the knee. New York: Churchill Livingstone, 1993:739–804

6. Whiteside LA, Milhalko WM. Surgical procedure for flexion contracture and recurvatum in total knee arthroplasty. Clin Orthop Relat Res 2002; (404):189–195

7. Rodriguez-Merchan EC. Instability following total knee arthroplasty. HSS J 2011;7(3):273–278

8. Baldini A, Castellani L, Traverso F, Balatri A, Balato G, Franceschini V. The difficult primary total knee arthroplasty: a review. Bone Joint J 2015; 97-B(10, Suppl A):30–39

9. Su EP. Fixed flexion deformity and total knee arthroplasty. J Bone Joint Surg Br 2012; 94(11, Suppl A):112–115

10. Shusaku M. Total knee arthroplasty in patients with genu recurvatum. Orthopaedic Proceedings 2016;98-B(Suppl 3):26–26

Computer-Navigated TKR for Extra-Articular Deformity

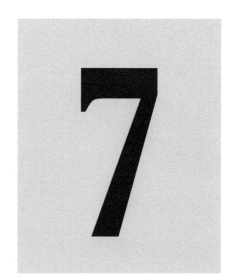

Anoop Jhurani and Piyush Agarwal

Introduction

- Extra-articular deformity is a secondary angulation below or above an arthritic knee which can significantly affect the deformity correction at the knee during total knee arthroplasty (TKA).
- Such deformities may result from malunions, stress fractures, pathological fractures, and other surgical procedures such as a high tibial osteotomy (HTO), distal femoral osteotomy (DFO), etc.[1]
- Metabolic bone disorders like Rickets, osteomalacia, Paget's disease may also result in coronal and sagittal plane deformities.
- The extra-articular deformities can present in any or all of the sagittal, coronal, or rotational planes.
- In conventional knee replacement surgery, cutting guides use intramedullary femoral instrumentation for executing the distal femoral cut and extramedullary tibial instrumentation for the proximal tibial cut.
- However, in patients with extra-articular deformities, it may be difficult or impossible to pass the intramedullary instruments in the right angle and direction. Hence, bony cut perpendicular to the mechanical axis may be difficult to obtain with the use of conventional instrumentation.[2]
- The resulting malaligned TKA components may lead to patellar maltracking, early aseptic loosening, and a higher rate of insert wear.[3]
- Navigation helps by avoiding the need to open the femoral canal and adjusting the bony cut appropriately in all three planes.
- This aids in achieving a measured resection with a graduated soft tissue releases to attain gap balance.
- Therefore, the patients with extra-articular deformities are ideal candidates for navigation-assisted total knee replacement (TKR) surgery.[4]

- To reconstruct such challenging knees, the surgeons are advocated to use navigation technology routinely in day-to-day practice.

Principle for Intra-Articular Correction of Extra-Articular Deformity

- The effect of extra-articular deformity on intra-articular correction is inversely proportional to its distance from the knee. Hence closer the extra-articular deformity to the knee, more profound its effect on intra-articular management during TKA[5,6] (**Fig. 7.1** and **Fig. 7.2**)
- The intra-articular correction of the extra-articular deformity is possible if the coronal plane deformity is 20 degrees or less in the femur and 30 degrees or less in tibia.[7] Deformities exceeding these limits require a corrective extra-articular osteotomy (staged or simultaneous).[8]
- The factors which should be considered to decide if an intra-articular correction is possible for an extra-articular deformity include:
  - Magnitude of deformity.
  - Distance of the deformity from the knee.
  - Direction/plane of the deformity.
  - Integrity of surrounding soft tissue structures.
  - Patient factors such as:
    - Age.
    - BMI.
    - Function (preoperative ambulatory status and knee range of motion [ROM]).
    - Bone quality.
    - Associated comorbidities.
- An intra-articular correction has the advantages of a single incision, lower incidence of anesthesia-related

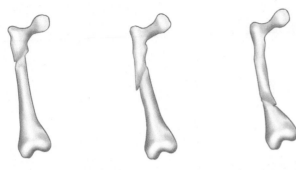

Fig. 7.1 Extra-articular deformity in femur. The closer the deformity to the knee, the more its effect on intra-articular correction.

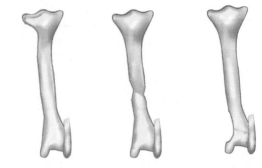

Fig. 7.2 Extra-articular deformity in tibia. The deformity can be in metaphysis, diaphysis, or near the ankle.

complications, and decreased wound-healing problems associated with osteotomies.

- A simultaneous corrective osteotomy can cause complications like wound dehiscence, decreased knee ROM, nonunion of osteotomy site, infection, arthrofibrosis, and pulmonary embolism.[1]

Case Illustrations

- Long bone bowing:
  - Varus bowing of femur and tibia.
  - Valgus bowing of femur and tibia.
- Extra articular deformity in femur:
  - Malunited proximal femur fracture.
  - Malunited diaphyseal femur fracture.
  - Malunited distal femur fracture.
- Extra articular deformity in tibia.
  - Malunited proximal tibia fracture (metaphyseal region).
  - Post-high tibial osteotomy (HTO):
    - ○ Medial open wedge osteotomy.
    - ○ Lateral closing wedge osteotomy.
    - ○ HTO with implant in situ.
  - Nonunion proximal tibia fracture (TKR with tibial extension rod).
  - Nonunion proximal tibia fracture (TKR with open reduction and internal fixation [ORIF]).
  - Malunited diaphyseal tibia fracture.
  - Malunited distal tibia fracture.
- Post proximal fibular osteotomy.

Long Bone Bowing

Varus Bowing of Femur and Tibia

- A 65-year-old lady presented with difficulty in walking for 4 years.
- Associated comorbidities were CAD, hypothyroidism, and diabetes mellitus.
- The patient was on oral Vitamin D and calcium supplements from the last 5 years for hypovitaminosis D (Serum Vitamin D = 20).

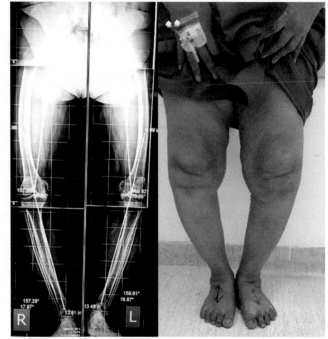

Fig. 7.3 Full-length lower limb radiograph and image of the patient.

- On examination, the patient had 25-degree varus deformity, knee ROM of 10 to 110 degrees and the knee was mediolaterally stable (**Fig. 7.3**).
- The preoperative full-length lower limb radiographs revealed femoral, tibial bowing, coxa vara, and low-neck shaft angle indicating constitutional varus deformity.[9] Such findings can't be appreciated with standard radiological films of knee with AP/lateral views (**Fig. 7.4**).
- The preoperative kinematics graph shows a severe uncorrectable varus deformity (**Fig. 7.5**).
- Constitutional varus is difficult to correct with bony cuts and soft tissue releases intra-articular as the deformity originates from bowed femur and tibia apart from the knee joint.

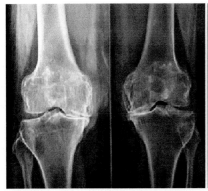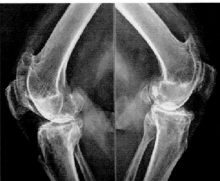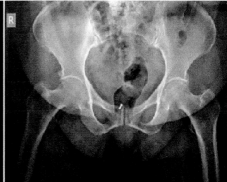

Fig. 7.4   Preoperative radiographs.

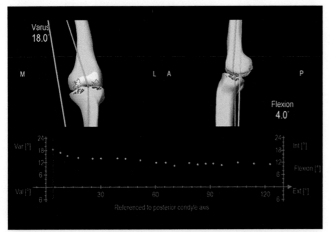

Fig. 7.5   Initial limb alignment and kinematics.

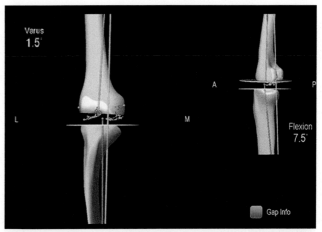

Fig. 7.6   3D model by navigation showing varus bowing,

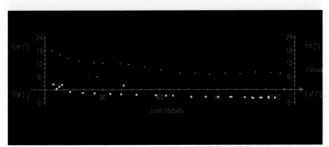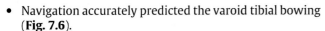

Fig. 7.7 Postoperative limb alignment and corrected kinematics.

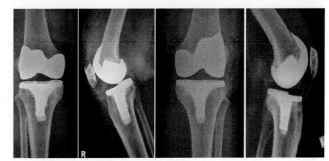

Fig. 7.8   Postoperative radiographs.

- Navigation accurately predicted the varoid tibial bowing (**Fig. 7.6**).
- Meticulous soft tissue balancing was essential to maintain optimal stability of the knee while restoring mechanical alignment of the lower limb.
- Severe varus deformity originating due to constitutional varus apart from the knee can be left in overall alignment of 2- to 3-degree varus as it is impossible to correct extra-articular varus at the knee joint without causing instability.
- The postoperative kinematics show complete correction of varus after cuts and releases (**Fig. 7.7**).

- Femoral and tibial prosthesis components in an acceptable position with a corrected limb alignment can be seen in postoperative radiographs (**Fig. 7.8**).

Pearls

- Bedridden patients should be evaluated for the presence of deep vein thrombosis (DVT) and/or stress fractures.
- X-rays of the pelvis with both hips should always be considered in such cases to exclude the presence of any stress fracture in the subtrochanteric region.

Pitfalls

- In cases with constitutional varus, it may be difficult to assess the residual deformity without the aid of navigation.
- Utilizing the conventional technique for performing TKA can result in residual malalignment and varus deformity.[10]

Valgus Tibial Bowing

- Valgoid deformity in tibia along with lateral compartment arthritis leading to an overall valgus alignment of the lower limb can be seen in preoperative radiographs (**Fig. 7.9**).

- These result mostly from metabolic disorders, skeletal dysplasia, or physeal trauma.[11]
- The preoperative kinematics graph demonstrates a valgus with recurvatum deformity which was correctable at ROM 90 degree and beyond (**Fig. 7.10**).
- Navigation accurately predicted the valgoid bowing in the tibia (**Fig. 7.11**).
- Mearsured distal femur and proximal tibia cut with popliteus pie crusting was done to balance the knee.
- Measured distal femur and proximal tibia cut with popliteus pie crusting was done to balance the knee.
- Complete correction of deformity in the sagittal and coronal planes can be seen on postoperative kinematics (**Fig. 7.12**).
- The postoperative radiographs show well-aligned components with corrected deformities (**Fig. 7.13**).

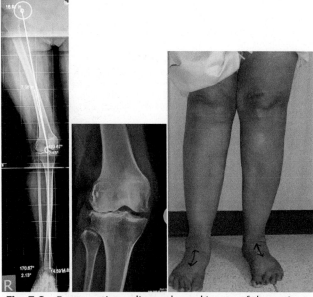

Fig. 7.9 Preoperative radiographs and image of the patient.

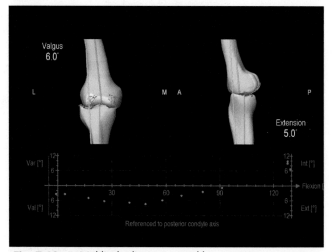

Fig. 7.10 Initial limb alignment and kinematics.

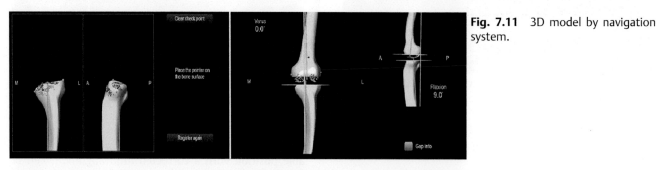

Fig. 7.11 3D model by navigation system.

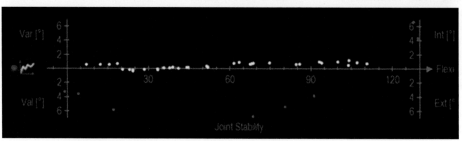

Fig. 7.12 Postoperative limb alignment and corrected kinematics.

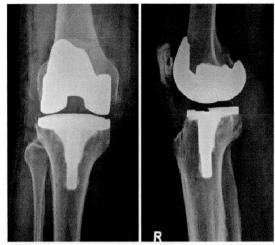

Fig. 7.13 Postoperative radiographs.

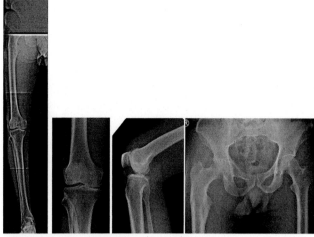

Fig. 7.14 Preoperative radiographs.

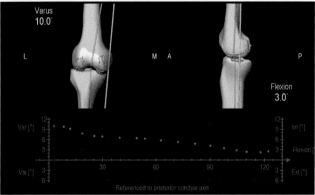

Fig. 7.15 Initial limb alignment and kinematics.

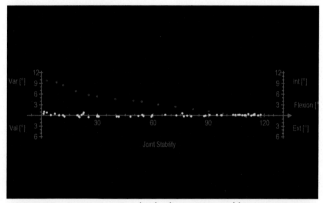

Fig. 7.16 Postoperative limb alignment and kinematics.

Extra-Articular Deformity in Femur

Malunited Proximal Femur Fracture

- The preoperative radiographs show malunited proximal femur (subtrochanteric) fracture and medial compartment osteoarthritis of the knee joint (**Fig. 7.14**).
- In this case, the malunion has a minimal impact on the intra-articular arthritic process of the knee. This makes it easier to correct such deformities in comparison to distal femoral fractures.
- The preoperative kinematic graph shows a 10-degree varus with a neutral sagittal plane alignment of the knee (**Fig. 7.15**).
- Under-resection of distal femur with mild posteromedial soft tissue release was done to correct varus deformity.
- The postoperative kinematics demonstrate the complete correction of the deformity (**Fig. 7.16**).
- Corrected limb alignment with well-placed prosthesis components are seen on postop X-rays (**Fig. 7.17**).

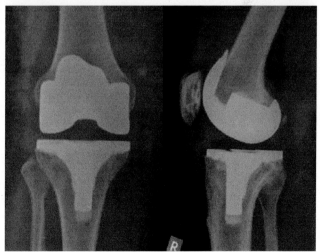

Fig. 7.17 Postoperative radiographs.

Pitfalls

- Proximal femoral malunion may be missed if surgery is planned only with standard small X-ray films of the knee joint.

Malunited Diaphyseal Femur Fracture

- A 50-year-old lady presented with complaints of pain in the left knee with a history of ipsilateral femur shaft fracture 35 years back which was managed conservatively with a hip spica cast.
- The patient was household ambulatory being able to walk 500 meters with a walker support.
- There was no tenderness, swelling, discharge, or sinus at the healed fracture site.
- Full length X-ray of femur show varus malunion in the femoral shaft with sagittal plane angulation. (**Fig. 7.18** and **Fig. 7.19**)

- Navigation shows severe varus flexion deformity with uncorrectable varus throughout ROM (**Fig. 7.20**).
- Angel wing can be used to check that DFC does not violate origin of lateral collateral ligament (**Fig. 7.21**).
- Reduction osteotomy of the tibia along with posteromedial soft tissue release was done to correct the deformity.
- Postoperative navigation screen showing complete correction of sagittal and coronal plane deformity (**Fig. 7.22**).
- The postoperative AP and lateral view radiographs demonstrate well-aligned prosthesis components in both coronal and sagittal planes. (**Fig. 7.23** and **Fig. 7.24**)

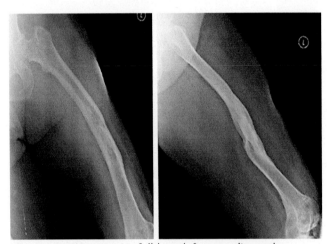

Fig. 7.18 Preoperative full-length femur radiographs

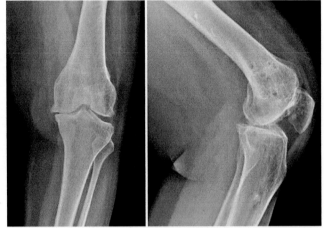

Fig. 7.19 Anteroposterior (AP) and lateral views of knee.

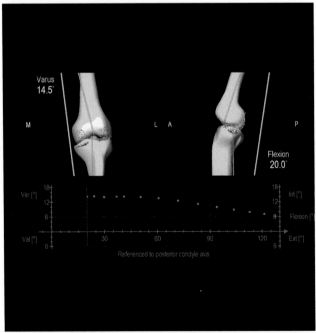

Fig. 7.20 Preoperative limb alignment and kinematics.

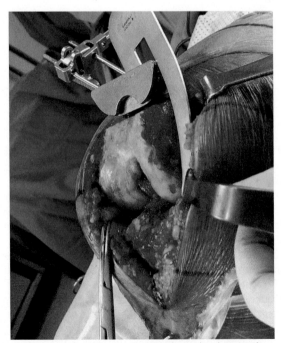

Fig. 7.21 Angel wing can be used to check DFC does not violate lateral collateral ligament (LCL).

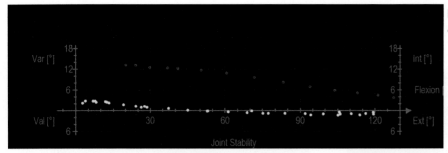

Fig. 7.22 Postoperative limb alignment and kinematics.

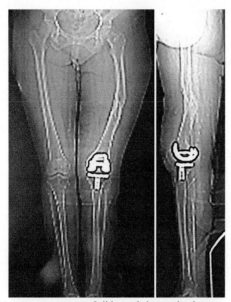

Fig. 7.23 Postoperative full length lower limb X-rays.

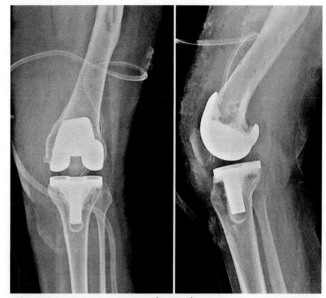

Fig. 7.24 Postoperative radiographs.

Malunited Distal Femoral Fracture

- This patient had sustained an open distal femur fracture a decade back which was managed elsewhere with ORIF and screw fixation.
- The hardware was removed 6 years back due to the complaints of pain at the screw sites.
- On examination, the patient had multiple healed scars around the knee from previous injury and surgical procedures.
- There was muscle wasting in the affected limb, with the overlying skin being nonadherent and mobile.
- The right knee ROM was 10 to 90 degrees, with no discharge or tenderness at the previously fractured site.
- The preoperative long-leg radiograph revealed a malunited distal femur metaphyseal fracture with a varus angulation (**Fig. 7.25**).
- The anteroposterior and lateral radiographic views of the knee show posttraumatic tricompartmental osteoarthritis with a malunited distal femur fracture.
- It is not possible to do conventional TKR in this case as intramedullary jig cannot be negotiated through malformed distal femur.

- The skin incision should be planned before proceeding with the surgery.
- The authors preferred a medial skin incision for achieving better closure in this case.
- Plastic surgery opinion can be taken in cases with a deficient soft tissue envelope (**Fig. 7.26**).

Pearls

- Whenever multiple prior incisions are present, it is advisable to use the most recent and/or lateral longitudinal incision.[12]
- In cases where the skin elasticity is lost or the prior incisions have made the skin immobile, thin, or adherent, tissue expanders can be utilized.
- If a new skin incision is planned, it should be at least two finger breadths (4 cm) away from the previous surgical scar marks.[13]
- The new incision should intersect an old incision at right angles only. If they intersect at an acute angle, it may increase the chances of skin necrosis at the wound edges.[13]

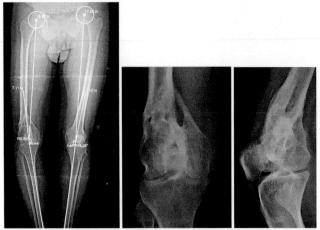

Fig. 7.25 Preoperative radiographs.

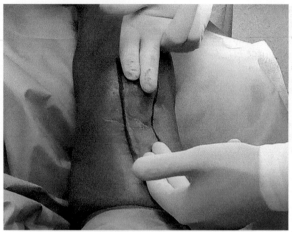

Fig. 7.26 Incision planning in total knee arthroplasty (TKA).

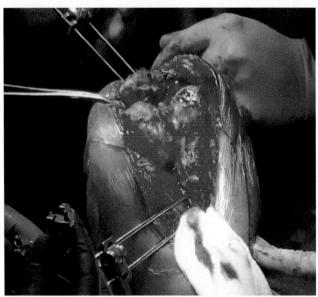

Fig. 7.27 Malformed distal femur with extensive scarring of quadriceps mechanism.

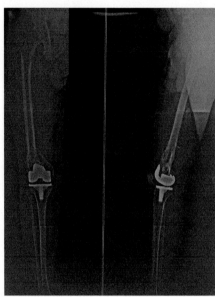

Fig. 7.28 Postoperative full-length lower limb radiographs.

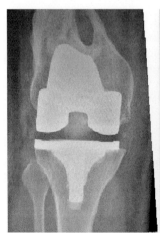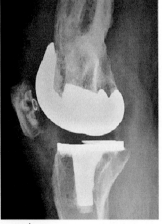

Fig. 7.29 Postoperative radiographs.

- The screws need to be placed proximal to the malunion site (**Fig. 7.27**).
- Exposure included rectus snip, clearance of lateral and medial gutters, intra-articular and suprapatellar fibrous tissue excision so as to mobilize the knee to perform the operation.
- A well-aligned mechanical axis and complete correction in the sagittal plane can be seen in postoperative AP and lateral view of long leg radiographs (**Fig. 7.28**).
- The postoperative AP and lateral views of the knee demonstrates well-aligned femoral and tibial prosthesis components (**Fig. 7.29**).

Pitfalls

- The diaphyseal Schanz screws can be a potential source for iatrogenic fractures.
- The pins should be unicortical to prevent stress riser effect.

Points to Remember

- Greater the deformity and proximity to the knee joint, more will be its impact on the intra-articular correction.[5]
- The femoral diaphyseal deformities greater than 20 degrees should be addressed separately from TKA. Intra-articular corrections of such deformities at the time of the TKA may lead to large asymmetrical cuts, damage to collaterals, and instability.[1]
- The femoral osteotomy can be performed simultaneously with TKA or as a staged procedure. The choices of fixation of the osteotomy include a plate and an intramedullary stem, a blade plate without an intramedullary stem, or a long-stem, press-fit, femoral prosthesis.

Extra-Articular Deformity in Tibia

Principles

- An intra-articular correction of the extra-articular deformity is possible if the coronal plane deformity is 30 degrees or less in the tibia.[1]
- The treatment of an extra-articular (EA) deformity of the tibia with a single-stage intra-articular (IA) correction is the preferred intervention when performing TKA, as an extra-articular osteotomy delays the recovery and increases the risk of postoperative complications.
- Preoperative planning is essential for an IA correction of an EA deformity to ensure that the tibial bone cut does not violate the insertion of the collateral ligaments.
- With a more significant deformity, relative over-resection of the lateral tibia (in a varus knee) or the medial tibia (in a valgus knee) can create relative laxity on the side of overresection. This creates a paradoxical situation causing mediolateral gap imbalance. Such cases can be managed with PS plus or constrained inserts.
- When an IA correction of an EA deformity is not possible, a staged or simultaneous correction of EA deformity is done to normalize the tibial resection during the same sitting or subsequently done TKR.

Malunited Proximal Tibial Fracture (Metaphyseal Region)

- A 60-year-old gentleman presented with difficulty in walking and pain in the right knee for 1 year.

- The patient had a history of trauma 10 years back when he sustained a proximal tibial fracture which was managed conservatively with splint support.
- There was no swelling, scar mark, sinuses, or redness at the operative site.
- The medial joint line of the knee joint was tender with no instability in the mediolateral plane.
- The knee ROM was 15-degree hyperextension to 120 degrees of flexion.
- The preoperative radiographs of the right lower limb show a malunited proximal tibial fracture (**Fig. 7.30**).
- There was reversal of normal slope and recurvatum deformity in the weight-bearing lateral view of the lower limb radiograph (**Fig. 7.31**).
- The anteroposterior and lateral views of the knee demonstrate posttraumatic arthritis and anterior sloping tibial plateau due to the malunited proximal tibial fracture (**Fig. 7.32**).
- A severe recurvatum deformity (15 degree) with neutral coronal alignment can be seen in preoperative kinematic graph (**Fig. 7.33**).
- The verification of the distal femoral cut was performed (**Fig. 7.34**).
- The 3D image of proximal tibia correctly predicted the bone morphology and the reversed tibial slope (**Fig. 7.35**).
- A minimal tibial cut with a neutral tibial slope was planned to compensate for the loose flexion gap (**Fig. 7.36**).

Pearls

- The normal posterior tibial slope varies from 4 to 7 degrees.[14]
- The posterior tibial slope is positively correlated with the knee ROM especially in a CR knee as compared to a PS knee.[15]

- The postoperative kinematics show the correction of deformity in both sagittal and coronal plane (**Fig. 7.37**).
- The postoperative X-rays demonstrate a well-aligned TKA prosthesis (**Fig. 7.38**).

Pearls

- The authors prefer to recreate the natural tibial slope whenever possible.
- However, in cases with previous osteotomy or malunited fractures, minimal posterior slope or neutral slope can be planned to balance the flexion gap without compromising the knee ROM.[16]

Pitfalls

An excessive slope can lead to anterior dislocation of the tibia and other biomechanical changes in the knee resulting in early wear-off.[17]

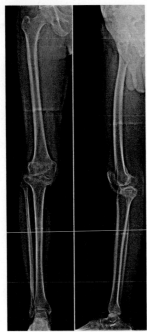

Fig. 7.30 Preoperative full-length lower limb radiographs.

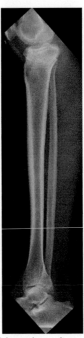

Fig. 7.31 Tibial full-length radiograph showing anterior tibial slope.

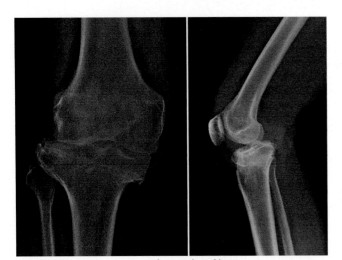

Fig. 7.32 Preoperative radiographs of knee.

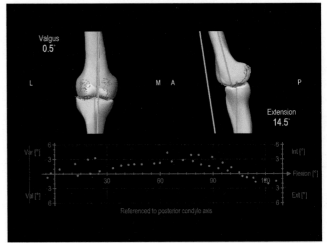

Fig. 7.33 Initial limb alignment and kinematics.

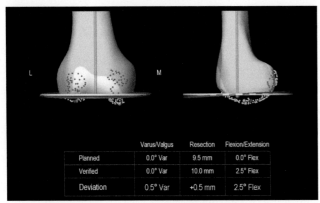

Fig. 7.34 Distal femur cut verification.

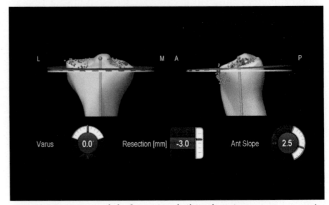

Fig. 7.35 3D model of proximal tibia showing posttraumatic defect.

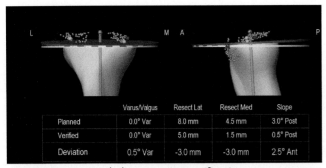

Fig. 7.36 Proximal tibia resection verification.

	Varus/Valgus	Resect Lat	Resect Med	Slope
Planned	0.0° Var	8.0 mm	4.5 mm	3.0° Post
Verified	0.0° Var	5.0 mm	1.5 mm	0.5° Post
Deviation	0.5° Var	-3.0 mm	-3.0 mm	2.5° Ant

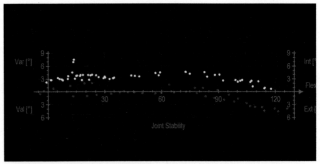

Fig. 7.37 Postoperative limb alignment and kinematics.

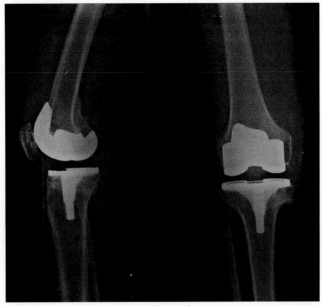

Fig. 7.38 Postoperative radiographs.

Post–High Tibial Osteotomy (HTO)

- HTO is advocated for the patients with early medial compartment osteoarthritis associated with varus alignment.
- It is usually performed in young patients, <50 years of age, having good cartilage stock.
- It corrects the weight-bearing axis, resulting in decreased stress over the involved joint compartment.[18]
- In most cases, the results deteriorate with time and may require conversion to a TKA.[19]
- It is challenging to manage such cases due to the history of previous knee surgery.
- Studies have revealed an increased revision and complication rates in patients undergoing TKA after an HTO.[19]
- A previous HTO makes TKA technically more demanding because of scar marks, anatomical distortion of tibial metaphysis, and alteration of tibial slope.[20]
- Lateral closed-wedge osteotomy causes proximation of the tibial tuberosity to the joint line due to wedge resection, resulting in patella alta. However, most cases present as patella baja because of postoperative immobilization and scarring. It also results in decreased posterior slope or reversal of slope.[21]
- Medial open-wedge osteotomy increases the posterior tibial slope and causes shortening of the patellar tendon, which presents as patella baja.[19]
- Osteotomy with an implant in situ may need an additional incision or surgery for implant removal.
- Navigation helps in overcoming these manifestations and in balancing the gaps with minimal soft tissue release.[18]
- It also guides in the correction of the tibial slope with the restoration of the normal joint line.

Navigated TKA Post-Medial Open-Wedge Osteotomy

- A 60-year-old gentleman presented with complaints of pain in the right knee for 2 years.
- The patient had a history of an HTO done 7 years back. The impinging implants were removed 6 months back.
- On examination, there was 25-degree varus and 15 degree of fixed flexion deformity with ROM of 15 to 120 degrees.

- An extra-articular proximal tibial deformity post-HTO with an arthritic right knee can be seen in full-length lower limb AP and lateral radiographs (**Fig. 7.39**).
- The navigation graph shows a fixed uncorrectable varus (22 degrees) and flexion deformity (13 degrees) (**Fig. 7.40**)
- The distal femoral cut verification navigation values elicit additional cut planned for correction of the flexion deformity (**Fig. 7.41**).
- An 11-mm cut from the lateral tibial condyle with almost no bone being resected from the medial tibial condyle (**Fig. 7.42**).
- This large lateral cut opened the lateral space both in extension and flexion causing relative instability. This needs to be balanced by significant medial releases or a constrained insert.

- Complete correction of the flexion and varus deformity seen in final kinematic graph (**Fig. 7.43**).
- The postoperative radiographs and scanogram of this patient confirmed the accurate alignment of the prosthetic components and the complete correction of the deformity (**Fig. 7.44**).

- The tibial mechanical axis shifts medially or antero-medially after HTO, which can cause the tibial prosthesis stem to hit against the lateral tibial cortex. The tibial component should be undersized, medially placed, or offset stem can be used to prevent this complication.[22]

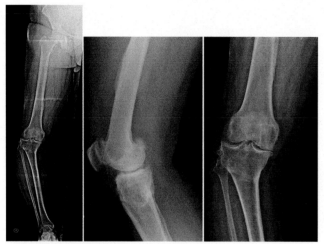

Fig. 7.39 Preoperative radiographs.

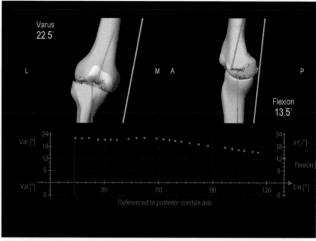

Fig. 7.40 Preoperative limb alignment and kinematics.

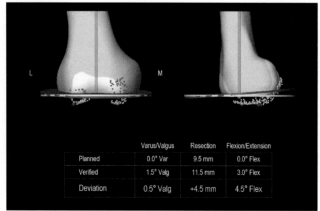

Fig. 7.41 Distal femur cut verification.

	Varus/Valgus	Resection	Flexion/Extension
Planned	0.0° Var	9.5 mm	0.0° Flex
Verified	1.5° Valg	11.5 mm	3.0° Flex
Deviation	0.5° Valg	+4.5 mm	4.5° Flex

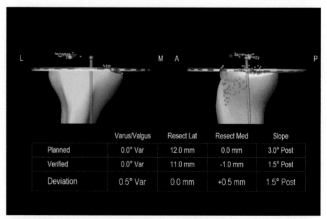

Fig. 7.42 Proximal tibia cut verification.

	Varus/Valgus	Resect Lat	Resect Med	Slope
Planned	0.0° Var	12.0 mm	0.0 mm	3.0° Post
Verified	0.0° Var	11.0 mm	-1.0 mm	1.5° Post
Deviation	0.5° Var	0.0 mm	+0.5 mm	1.5° Post

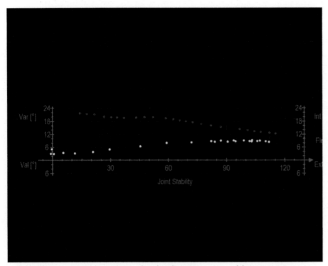

Fig. 7.43 Postoperative limb alignment and kinematics.

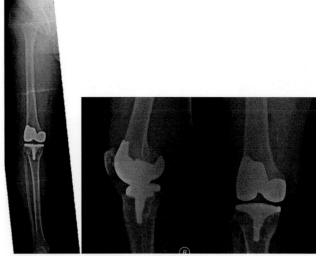

Fig. 7.44 Postoperative radiographs.

Lateral Closed-Wedge Osteotomy of the Proximal Tibia

- A 50-year-old gentleman presented with complaints of pain in the right knee and difficulty in walking for 1 year.
- He had undergone a lateral closed-wedge osteotomy 10 years back for similar complaints.
- There were no signs of infection and swelling at the previous operative site.
- A healed surgical scar was present over the lateral side of the tibial tuberosity.
- On examination there was 5-degree varus deformity with knee ROM 0 to 120 degrees.
- The preoperative radiographs show post-HTO arthritic knee with varus alignment and reduced tibial slope (**Fig. 7.45**).
- The preoperative kinematic analysis demonstrates a varus deformity with neutral sagittal alignment (**Fig. 7.46**).
- An underresection of the distal femur was performed as such knees tend to become loose in extension after the tibial cut (**Fig. 7.47**)
- Underresection of the proximal tibia was planned with a neutral slope to balance the flexion gap (**Fig. 7.48**).

- A neutral slope is still perpendicular to the mechanical axis in sagittal plane, considering that the tibial plateau is upsloped post HTO (**Fig. 7.49**).
- Mild posteromedial soft tissue was done to correct the varus deformity.
- The postoperative kinematic graph elicits balanced mediolateral gaps with correction of the deformity (**Fig. 7.50**).
- Well-aligned components with corrected limb alignment can be seen in postoperative radiographs (**Fig. 7.51**).

Pearls

- In patients with the presence of multiple scar marks over the knee joint, the surgical incision is preferred over the most lateral scar as the lateral flap is more vulnerable to necrosis because most of the blood supply and lymphatic drainage originates on the medial side.[20]
- In cases with patellar scarring, the patella may be difficult to evert. Stepwise soft tissue release, rectus snip, or rarely tibial tuberosity osteotomy (TTO) may be required.

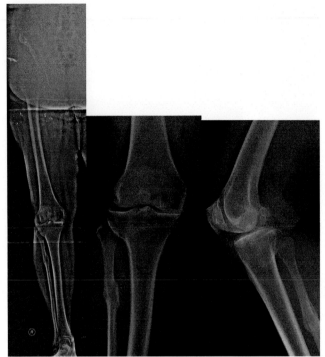

Fig. 7.45 Preoperative radiographs.

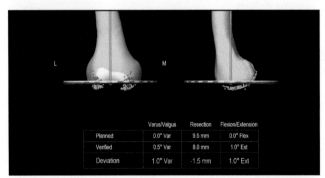

	Varus/Valgus	Resection	Flexion/Extension
Planned	0.0° Var	9.5 mm	0.0° Flex
Verified	0.5° Var	8.0 mm	1.0° Ext
Deviation	1.0° Var	-1.5 mm	1.0° Ext

Fig. 7.47 Distal femur cut verification.

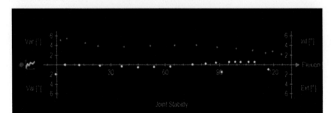

	Varus/Valgus	Resect Med	Resect Lat	Slope
Planned	0.0° Var	8.0 mm	7.5 mm	3.0° Post
Verified	0.5° Var	5.5 mm	4.5 mm	2.5° Post
Deviation	0.0° Var	+0.5 mm	+0.5 mm	4.0° Ant

Fig. 7.48 Proximal tibia cut verification.

Fig. 7.50 Postoperative limb alignment and kinematics.

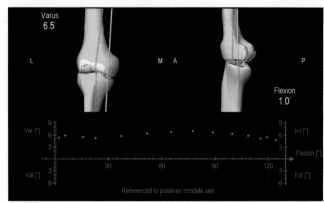

Fig. 7.46 Preoperative limb alignment and kinematics.

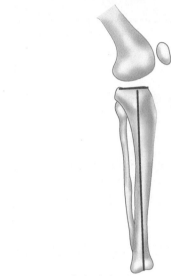

Fig. 7.49 Neutral tibial slope.

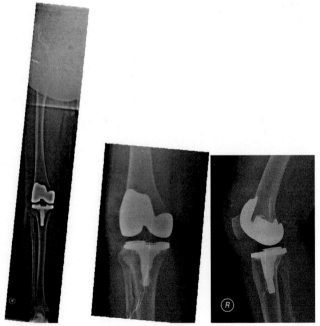

Fig. 7.51 Postoperative radiographs.

HTO with an Implant in situ

- A 65-year-old lady presented with complaints of pain and difficulty walking for 6 months.
- The patient had a history of a lateral closed-wedge HTO with staple fixation in right knee, 8 years back.
- There were no signs of infection and swelling at the previous operative site.
- The staple was palpable under the skin laterally and the knee had 10 degrees of valgus deformity with ROM of 0 to 120 degrees.
- The preoperative radiographs show tricompartmental osteoarthritis of the right knee joint with staple in the lateral condyle of tibia at the healed osteotomy site (**Fig. 7.52** and **Fig. 7.53**).

- The preoperative kinematic graph shows 10 degrees of valgus with neutral sagittal plane alignment (**Fig. 7.54**).
- The hardware from the previous surgery was removed at the time of surgical exposure of the knee through a separate small incision placed over the staple.
- Complete correction of deformity with 5 degrees of residual flexion seen in postoperative kinematic (**Fig. 7.55**).
- Minimal bone resection along with lateral soft tissue release to correct the valgus deformity was done to achieve appropriate limb alignment and ligament balance.
- The postoperative radiographs demonstrate corrected deformity with well-aligned prosthesis components (**Fig. 7.56**).

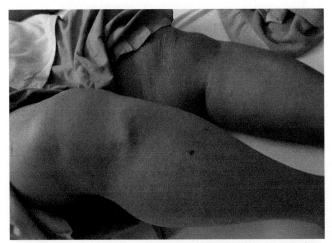

Fig. 7.52 Image of the knee showing implant puckering skin.

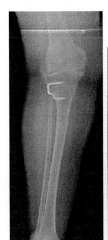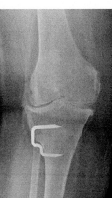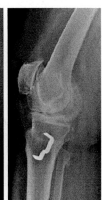

Fig. 7.53 Preoperative radiographs.

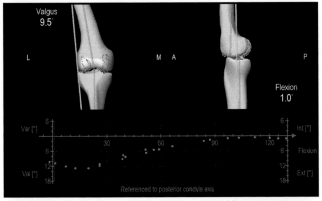

Fig. 7.54 Preoperative limb alignment and kinematics.

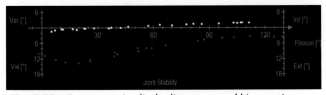

Fig. 7.55 Postoperative limb alignment and kinematics.

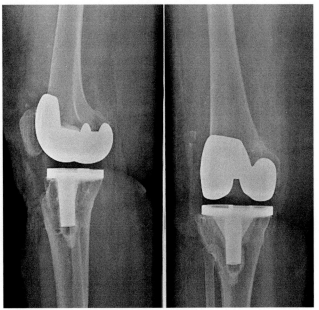

Fig. 7.56 Postoperative radiographs.

- It is recommended to resurface the patella in such cases, as the change in patellar height and peripatellar soft tissue scarring can affect the patellar tracking.[23]
- Meticulous lateral retinaculum release may be required for appropriate patellar tracking.

Nonunion Proximal Tibia Fracture (TKR with Tibial Extension Rod)

- A 50-year-old lady presented with inability to walk independently from last 6 months.
- The patient was a known case of rheumatoid arthritis.
- On examination, there was mild swelling, tenderness, and minimal abnormal mobility at the nonunion site present at the metaphyseal-diaphyseal junction of the left tibia.
- There was 25-degree varus deformity with 40 degrees of fixed flexion deformity (FFD) at the knee joint with further flexion to 120 degrees (**Fig. 7.57**).
- The full-length radiograph shows a varus alignment of the left lower limb at the nonunion site (**Fig. 7.58**).
- Absent intra-articular space, diffuse osteopenia, tricompartmental osteoarthritis, and nonunion of the proximal tibia shaft can be seen in preoperative radiographs.
- The fibula was intact causing relative immobility at the nonunion site.

- The tibial Schanz screws were placed distally in the tibia, away from the nonunion site (**Fig. 7.59**).
- Preoperative knee kinematics showed 23 degrees of uncorrectable varus and 36 degrees FFD (**Fig. 7.60**).
- The initial step during surgery was to perform a fibular osteotomy in the diaphyseal region (**Fig. 7.61**).
- Thereafter, the tibial nonunion site was meticulously exposed and an osteotomy was performed with a sharp 10-mm osteotome while protecting the pes anserinus insertion.
- The osteotomy site was reduced and secured with the help of a laminar spreader.
- A drill bit was passed to identify the tibial intramedullary canal under an image intensifier guidance (**Fig. 7.62**).
- Sequential reaming was done after the guide wire insertion in the intramedullary canal of the tibia.
- Trial stem was checked under C-arm to see that it is centrally positioned in AP and lateral views.
- Extra-articular osteotomy aided in correction of severe varus flexion as majority of the deformity was at the non union site.
- An additional distal femoral resection was planned to gain the extension space (**Fig. 7.63**).
- The external rotation of the femoral component was increased to open up the medial space in flexion so as to aid in balance of the mediolateral gap in flexion (**Fig. 7.64**).
- The postoperative navigation graph shows the correction of varus and flexion deformities (**Fig. 7.65**).
- The tibial osteotomy site was filled with the bone graft (**Fig. 7.66**).
- Well-aligned femoral and tibial components can be seen in postoperative radiographs (**Fig. 7.67**).
- The tibial extension rod secured rigid fixation in the tibial diaphysis, bypassing the nonunion site and obviating the need for any further internal fixation.

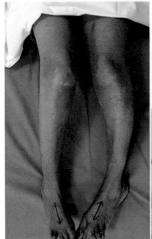
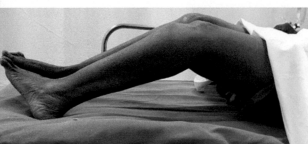

Fig. 7.57 Images of the bedridden patient.

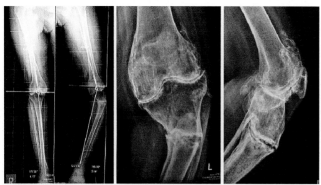

Fig. 7.58 Preoperative radiographs.

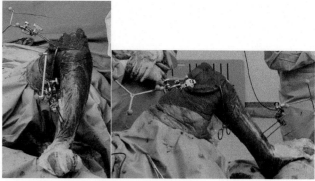

Fig. 7.59 Diaphyseal array placement.

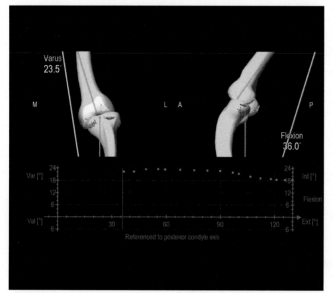

Fig. 7.60 Preoperative limb alignment and kinematics.

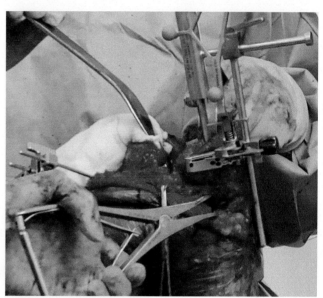

Fig. 7.61 Picture showing technique for correction of extra-articular deformity.

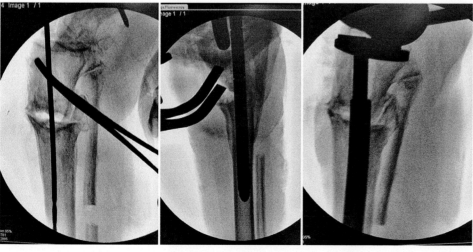

Fig. 7.62 Intraoperative image intensifier (IITV) images.

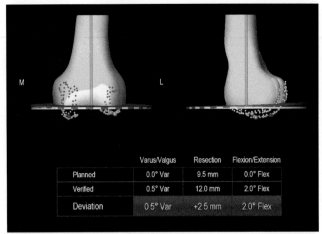

	Varus/Valgus	Resection	Flexion/Extension
Planned	0.0° Var	9.5 mm	0.0° Flex
Verified	0.5° Var	12.0 mm	2.0° Flex
Deviation	0.5° Var	+2.5 mm	2.0° Flex

Fig. 7.63 Distal femur cut verification.

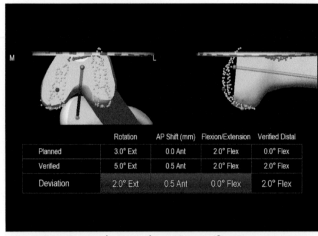

	Rotation	AP Shift (mm)	Flexion/Extension	Verified Distal
Planned	3.0° Ext	0.0 Ant	2.0° Flex	0.0° Flex
Verified	5.0° Ext	0.5 Ant	2.0° Flex	2.0° Flex
Deviation	2.0° Ext	0.5 Ant	0.0° Flex	2.0° Flex

Fig. 7.64 Femoral external rotation verification.

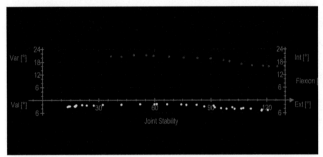

Fig. 7.65 Postoperative kinematics and limb alignment.

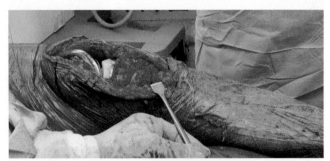

Fig. 7.66 Picture showing bone graft at osteotomy site.

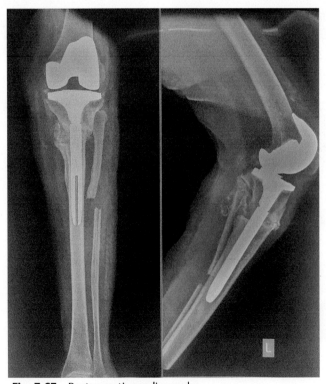

Fig. 7.67 Postoperative radiographs.

Nonunion of Proximal Tibia Fracture (TKR with ORIF)

- A 60-year-old woman presented with complaints of pain in the right knee and difficulty walking for the last 3 months.
- She was unable to bear weight over the affected leg for the past 1 week.
- On physical examination, swelling and tenderness with minimal abnormal mobility was present at the proximal tibia fracture site.
- The right knee was in 10-degree varus deformity and 10-degree FFD with further flexion to 120 degrees.
- Stress fracture at the proximal metaphyseal-diaphyseal junction of right tibia seen in preoperative X-ray (**Fig. 7.68**)

- Preoperative navigation screen shows moderate varus (12 degree) with mild flexion deformity (6.5 degree) (**Fig. 7.69**).
- To correct the varus flexion deformity, reduction osteotomy of the tibia along with posteromedial soft tissue release was done.
- Complete correction of deformity seen in postoperative navigation screen (**Fig. 7.70**).
- The postoperative X-rays show optimal alignment with well fixed prosthesis (**Fig. 7.71**).
- There was residual mobility at the fracture site after inserting the tibial prosthesis with an extension rod. Hence additional internal fixation with medial locking compression plate (LCP) was added making the construct stable.

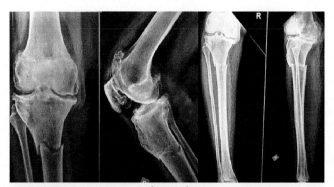

Fig. 7.68 Preoperative radiographs.

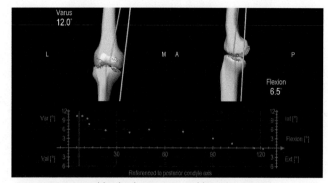

Fig. 7.69 Initial limb alignment and kinematics.

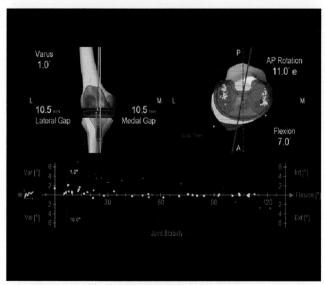

Fig. 7.70 Final limb alignment and kinematics.

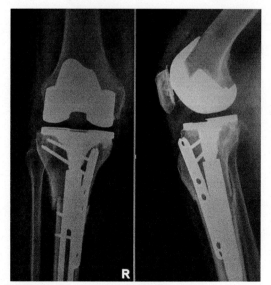

Fig. 7.71 Postoperative radiographs.

Malunited Diaphyseal Tibia Fracture

- A 55-year-old man presented with complaints of difficulty in walking and pain in both knees for 1 year.
- He had a history of left tibia shaft fracture 15 years back, which was managed conservatively elsewhere.
- On examination, there was no swelling, tenderness, scar mark, or discharge at the previously fractured site.
- There were 10-degree valgus and 5.5-degree recurvatum in sagittal plane of the left knee with further flexion to 130 degrees.

- The preoperative radiographs show tricompartmental osteoarthritis of the left knee with diaphyseal malunion of the left tibia (**Fig. 7.72** to **Fig. 7.74**).
- 10-degree correctable valgus with 5.5-degree recurvatum in sagittal plane seen in preoperative kinematic analysis (**Fig. 7.75**)
- A 10-mm distal femur bone resection was verified (**Fig. 7.76**).
- A minimal proximal tibial cut was planned, 2 mm from the lateral tibial condyle and 0 mm from the medial condyle of the tibia with 4 degrees of posterior slope (**Fig. 7.77**).
- The final kinematic analysis shows the uncorrected deformities in both the coronal and sagittal planes (**Fig. 7.78**).
- Gaps were found to be imbalanced more in flexion than extension.
- There was more than 2mm of gap imbalance in flexion with medial side opening more even after lateral soft tissue release.
- Semiconstrained insert was used to manage mild instability.
- The postoperative full-length leg view shows a complete correction of the mechanical alignment and satisfactory prosthesis positioning (**Fig. 7.79** and **Fig. 7.80**).

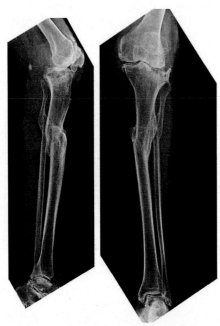

Fig. 7.72 Anteroposterior (AP) and lateral full-length tibia radiographs.

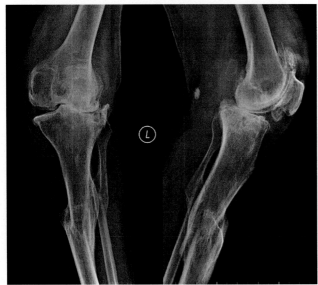

Fig. 7.73 Preoperative radiographs.

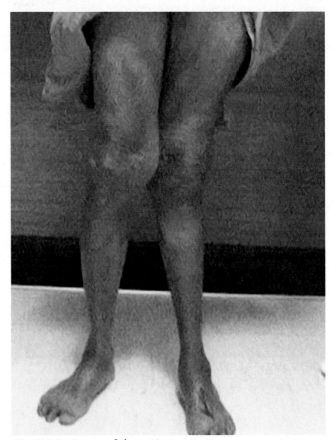

Fig. 7.74 Image of the patient.

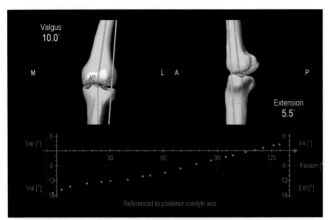

Fig. 7.75 Initial limb alignment and kinematics.

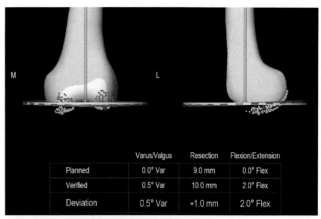

	Varus/Valgus	Resection	Flexion/Extension
Planned	0.0° Var	9.0 mm	0.0° Flex
Verified	0.5° Var	10.0 mm	2.0° Flex
Deviation	0.5° Var	+1.0 mm	2.0° Flex

Fig. 7.76 Distal femur cut verification.

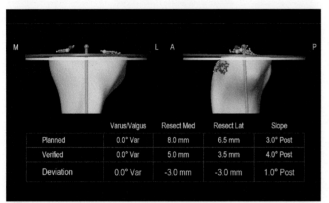

	Varus/Valgus	Resect Med	Resect Lat	Slope
Planned	0.0° Var	8.0 mm	6.5 mm	3.0° Post
Verified	0.0° Var	5.0 mm	3.5 mm	4.0° Post
Deviation	0.0° Var	-3.0 mm	-3.0 mm	1.0° Post

Fig. 7.77 Proximal tibia cut verification.

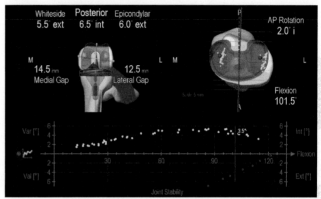

Fig. 7.78 Postoperative limb alignment and kinematics.

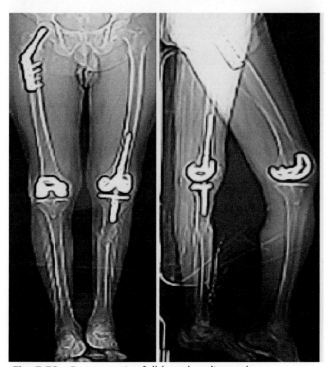

Fig. 7.79 Postoperative full-length radiographs

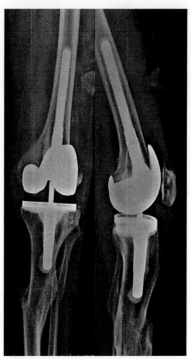

Fig. 7.80 Postoperative radiograph.

Malunited Distal Tibia Fracture

- A 50-year-old gentleman presented with complaints of pain in the left knee and difficulty in walking.
- The patient had a history of left distal tibia fracture 10 years back which was managed conservatively with a Patellar tendon bearing (PTB) cast elsewhere.
- There was no tenderness, swelling, discharge, or sinus.
- The left knee had varus–flexion deformity with further flexion to 110 degrees.
- The preoperative radiographs show osteoarthritis of the left knee with a malunited distal tibia fracture (**Fig. 7.81**).

- The presence of a deformity away from the knee joint has a minimal impact over the intra-articular correction.[5]
- Mild biplanar deformity of 7-degree varus and 4-degree flexion seen on preoperative kinematics (**Fig. 7.82**).
- A neutral tibial slope was planned to compensate for the procurvatum at the fracture site.
- The postoperative kinematic graph illustrated the correction of the biplanar deformity (**Fig. 7.83**).
- The postoperative radiographs show the correction of deformity with a well-aligned prosthesis (**Fig. 7.84**).

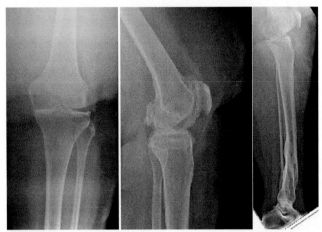

Fig. 7.81 Preoperative radiographs.

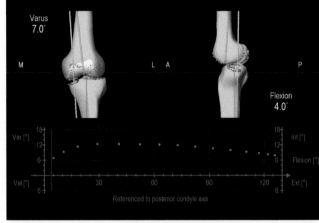

Fig. 7.82 Initial limb alignment and verification.

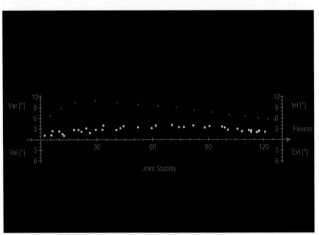

Fig. 7.83 Postoperative limb alignment and kinematics.

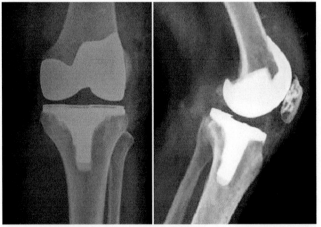

Fig. 7.84 Postoperative radiographs.

Malunited Proximal Femur and Distal Tibia Fracture

- A 62-year-old teacher presented with osteoarthritis of the right knee with history of right proximal femur fracture 10 years back and right distal tibia fracture 5 years back which were managed conservatively.
- On examination, there were no tenderness, swelling, discharge, or sinus at the previous fracture site.
- The right knee had 10-degree varus and 15-degree FFD with further flexion to 120 degrees.

- Patient had true shortening of 3 cm in right lower limb.
- Preoperative radiographs showing bone on bone arthritis causing pain and difficulty in walking (**Fig. 7.85** and **Fig. 7.86**).
- Careful history and examination may reveal old malunited fractures.
- They should be throughly evaluated to rule out nonunion or infection.
- Multiple fracture in same limb may cause true shortening which won't be corrected by TKA.
- Patient should be counseled regarding increasing shoe height to compensate for the shortening (**Fig. 7.87**).
- There was 4 degree of uncorrectable varus with 12 degree of FFD on preoperative knee kinematics. (**Fig. 7.88**)
- Near-normal distal femur resection was done as correction of mild varus would correct some flexion (**Fig. 7.89**).
- Posteromedial soft tissue release and reduction osteotomy were done to correct the varus–flexion deformity.
- 7 to 8 mm proximal tibia was resected to create space for minimal insert (9mm) (**Fig. 7.90**).

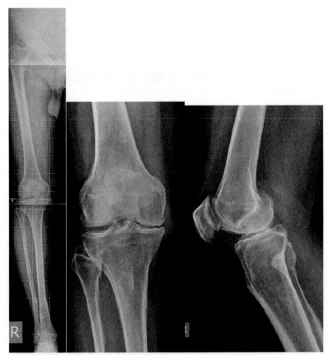

Fig. 7.85   Preoperative radiographs

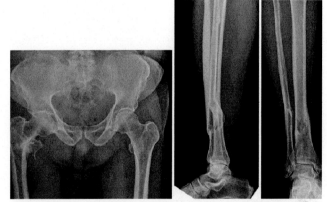

Fig. 7.86   Malunited proximal femur and distal tibia fracture.

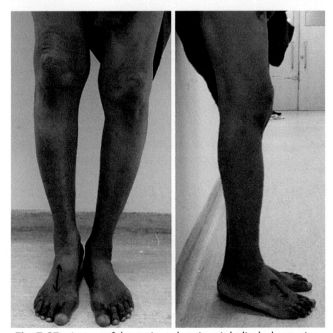

Fig. 7.87   Image of the patient showing right limb shortening.

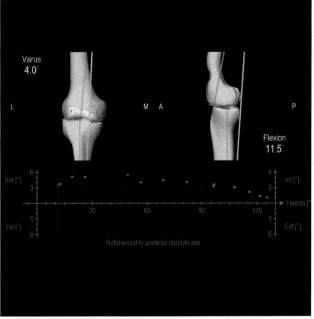

Fig. 7.88   Initial limb alignment and kinematics.

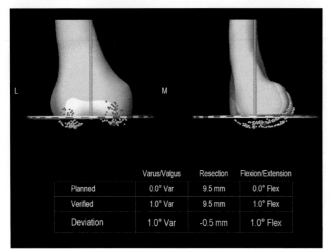

Fig. 7.89 Distal femur cut resection.

	Varus/Valgus	Resection	Flexion/Extension
Planned	0.0° Var	9.5 mm	0.0° Flex
Verified	1.0° Var	9.5 mm	1.0° Flex
Deviation	1.0° Var	-0.5 mm	1.0° Flex

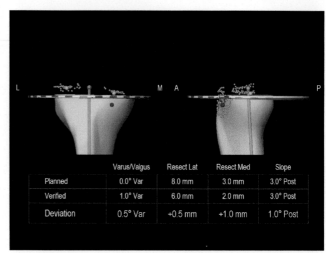

Fig. 7.90 Proximal tibia cut verification.

	Varus/Valgus	Resect Lat	Resect Med	Slope
Planned	0.0° Var	8.0 mm	3.0 mm	3.0° Post
Verified	1.0° Var	6.0 mm	2.0 mm	3.0° Post
Deviation	0.5° Var	+0.5 mm	+1.0 mm	1.0° Post

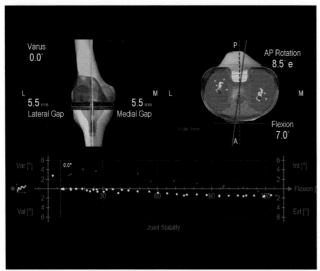

Fig. 7.91 Postoperative limb alignment and corrected kinematics.

- Postoperative kinematics shows complete correction of biplanar deformity with correction of knee alignment throughout ROM (**Fig. 7.91**).
- Complete correction of deformity with well-aligned and fixed knee component can be seen on postoperative radiographs (**Fig. 7.92**).

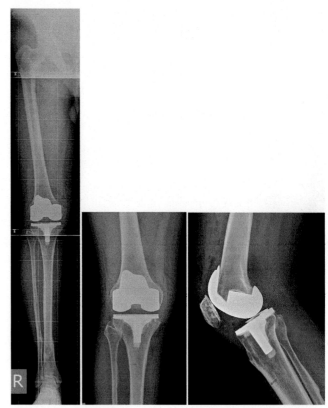

Fig. 7.92 Postoperative radiographs.

Points to Remember

- Long leg standing X-rays should always be obtained in cases with extra-articular deformity.
- Preoperative planning should include complete radiological evaluation like full-length standing X-ray, pelvis with both hips—AP, Knee—AP and lateral views, and soft tissue evaluation.
- CT scan may be advised for assessing the rotational malalignment at the extra-articular deformity.

Postproximal Fibular Osteotomy (PFO)

- Proximal fibular osteotomy is a relatively new treatment option advocated for the management of early medial compartment osteoarthritis.[24]
- This procedure is becoming popular in countries like India, China, and South Korea.[25]
- PFO is inexpensive, technically easy to perform and requires less rehabilitation in comparison to HTO, UKA, or TKA.[23]

- In this procedure, around 1 to 2 cm of a fibular strut is removed, usually 6 to 10 cm distal to the head of fibula.[26]
- It is postulated that PFO shifts the weight-bearing axis away from the overloaded medial compartment, thus correcting the varus deformity and thereby decreasing the pain.[26]
- However, it can be considered as a sham or placebo procedure since it neither alters the mechanism of arthritis nor does it correct the malalignment of the knee joint.

Pitfalls

- The most common complication associated with PFO is a transient neural injury to the branches of common peroneal nerve.[27]
- Navigation in such cases helps in the documentation of the deformity present and its correction intraoperatively.

- A 70-year-old woman presented with complaints of pain in the knee joint and difficulty in walking.
- The patient had undergone PFO on the left leg 6 months back but the pain persisted postsurgery.
- On examination, knee had varus flexion deformity with further flexion till 130 degrees.

- A varus alignment of the left lower limb with bone on bone arthritis in the medial compartment can be seen in preoperative radiographs. (**Fig. 7.93**).
- Evidence of previous PFO surgery is also noted.
- The intraoperative image showing completely worn-off cartilage over the medial femoral and tibial condyle (**Fig. 7.94**).
- The preoperative kinematic graph illustrated the biplanar deformity of the knee joint with 5-degrees of varus and 7-degrees of flexion (**Fig. 7.95**).
- Removal of osteophytes with minimal soft tissue releases corrected this mild deformity.

Pearls

- The patients should be examined thoroughly before surgery, especially for signs of peroneal nerve injury.
- Accurate documentation of the deformity aids in its correction during the surgery, along with being an important medicolegal record.

- The postoperative navigation kinematics graph shows the correction of the biplanar deformity with balanced gaps (**Fig. 7.96**).
- Restored mechanical alignment with a well-fixed prosthesis can be seen in postoperative radiographs (**Fig. 7.97**).

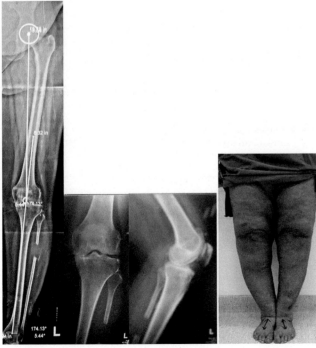

Fig. 7.93 Preoperative radiographs.

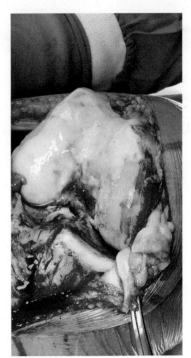

Fig. 7.94 Knee with complete loss of cartilage.

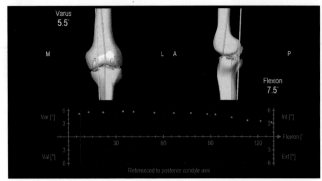

Fig. 7.95 Preoperative limb alignment and kinematics.

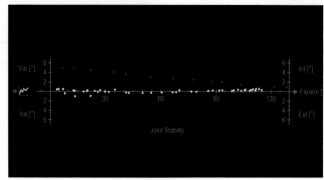

Fig. 7.96 Postoperative limb alignment and kinematics.

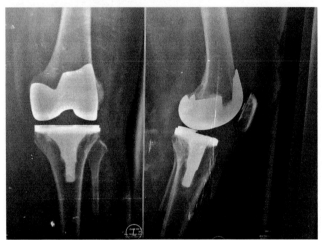

Fig. 7.97 Postoperative radiographs.

Points to Remember

- Always obtain long-leg standing X-ray films.
- Measure the magnitude of the extra-articular deformity preoperatively and confirm it intraoperatively.
- Estimate the distance of the extra-articular deformity from the knee joint.
- Determine the exact location of deformity: intra-articular, metaphyseal, or diaphyseal. The closer the deformity is to knee joint, more is its impact on the knee joint deformity correction.
- About 20 degrees of extra-articular deformity can be corrected intra-articularly during TKA without violating the collaterals. If the deformity is greater than that and is accompanied with nonunion or severe ligamentous instability, then it is advisable to correct the extra-articular deformity before as a separate procedure or during TKA with extended fixation modalities.
- The authors prefer the use of a semi-constrained insert (high and broad central post) in cases with mild mediolateral instability.
- A constrained prosthesis should also be available in the inventory while operating such challenging cases.

References

1. Rajgopal A, Vasdev A, Dahiya V, Tyagi VC, Gupta H. Total knee arthroplasty in extra articular deformities: a series of 36 knees. Indian J Orthop 2013;47(1):35–39

2. Rhee SJ, Seo CH, Suh JT. Navigation-assisted total knee arthroplasty for patients with extra-articular deformity. Knee Surg Relat Res 2013;25(4):194–201

3. Abdelnasser MK, Elsherif ME, Bakr H, Mahran M, Othman MHM, Khalifa Y. All types of component malrotation affect the early patient-reported outcome measures after total knee arthroplasty. Knee Surg Relat Res 2019;31(1):5

4. Tigani D, Masetti G, Sabbioni G, Ben Ayad R, Filanti M, Fosco M. Computer-assisted surgery as indication of choice: total knee arthroplasty in case of retained hardware or extra-articular deformity. Int Orthop 2012;36(7):1379–1385

5. Wolff AM, Hungerford DS, Pepe CL. The effect of extraarticular varus and valgus deformity on total knee arthroplasty. Clin Orthop Relat Res 1991; (271):35–51

6. Hungerford DS. Extraarticular deformity is always correctable intraarticularly: to the contrary. Orthopedics 2009;32

7. Sculco PK, Kahlenberg CA, Fragomen AT, Rozbruch SR. Management of extra-articular deformity in the setting of total knee arthroplasty. J Am Acad Orthop Surg 2019;27(18):e819–e830

8. Mullaji A, Shetty GM. Computer-assisted total knee arthroplasty for arthritis with extra-articular deformity. J Arthroplasty 2009;24(8):1164–9.e1

9. Bellemans J, Colyn W, Vandenneucker H, Victor J. The Chitranjan Ranawat award: is neutral mechanical alignment normal for all patients? The concept of constitutional varus. Clin Orthop Relat Res 2012;470(1):45–53

10. Kim CW, Lee CR. Effects of femoral lateral bowing on coronal alignment and component position after total knee arthroplasty: a comparison of conventional and navigation-assisted surgery. Knee Surg Relat Res 2018;30(1):64–73

11. Espandar R, Mortazavi SM, Baghdadi T. Angular deformities of the lower limb in children. Asian J Sports Med 2010;1(1):46–53

12. Engh GA. Exposure options for revision total knee arthroplasty. In: Bono JV, Scott RD, eds. Revision total knee arthroplasty. New York, NY: Springer; 2005: 63–75

13. Younger AS, Duncan CP, Masri BA. Surgical exposures in revision total knee arthroplasty. J Am Acad Orthop Surg 1998;6(1):55–64

14. Adulkasem N, Rojanasthien S, Siripocaratana N, Limmahakhun S. Posterior tibial slope modification in osteoarthritis knees with different ACL conditions: Cadaveric study of fixed-bearing UKA. J Orthop Surg (Hong Kong) 2019;27(2):2309499019836286

15. Kim KH, Bin SI, Kim JM. The correlation between posterior tibial slope and maximal angle of flexion after total knee arthroplasty. Knee Surg Relat Res 2012;24(3):158–163

16. Khanna V, Sambandam SN, Ashraf M, Mounasamy V. Extra-articular deformities in arthritic knees—a grueling challenge for arthroplasty surgeons: An evidence-based update. Orthop Rev (Pavia) 2018;9(4):7374

17. Seo SS, Kim CW, Kim JH, Min YK. Clinical results associated with changes of posterior tibial slope in total knee arthroplasty. Knee Surg Relat Res 2013;25(1):25–29

18. Song SJ, Bae DK. Computer-assisted navigation in high tibial osteotomy. Clin Orthop Surg 2016;8(4):349–357

19. Song SJ, Bae DK, Kim KI, Lee CH. Conversion total knee arthroplasty after failed high tibial osteotomy. Knee Surg Relat Res 2016;28(2):89–98

20. Bae DK, Song SJ, Yoon KH. Total knee arthroplasty following closed wedge high tibial osteotomy. Int Orthop 2010;34(2):283–287

21. Cerciello S, Vasso M, Maffulli N, Neyret P, Corona K, Panni AS. Total knee arthroplasty after high tibial osteotomy. Orthopedics 2014;37(3):191–198

22. Nagamine R, Inoue S, Miura H, Matsuda S, Iwamoto Y. Femoral shaft bowing influences the correction angle for high tibial osteotomy. J Orthop Sci 2007;12(3):214–218

23. Amendola A, Bonasia DE. Results of high tibial osteotomy: review of the literature. Int Orthop 2010;34(2):155–160

24. Vaish A, Kumar Kathiriya Y, Vaishya R. A critical review of proximal fibular osteotomy for knee osteoarthritis. Arch Bone Jt Surg 2019;7(5):453–462

25. Shanmugasundaram S, Kambhampati SBS, Saseendar S. Proximal fibular osteotomy in the treatment of medial osteoarthritis of the knee: a narrative review of literature. Knee Surg Relat Res 2019;31(1):16

26. ZeYu Huang YN, Xu B, Shen B, Kraus VB, Pei FX. Evidence and mechanism by which upper partial fibulectomy improves knee biomechanics and decreases knee pain of osteoarthritis. J Orthop Res 2018;36:2099–2108

27. Ogbemudia AO, Umebese PFA, Bafor A, Igbinovia E, Ogbemudia PE. The level of fibula osteotomy and incidence of peroneal nerve palsy in proximal tibial osteotomy. J Surg Tech Case Rep 2010;2(1):17–19

Computer-Navigated TKR in Knees with Retained Hardware

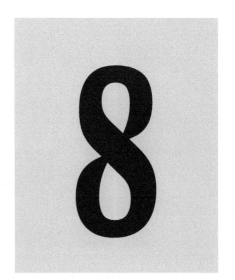

Anoop Jhurani and Piyush Agarwal

Introduction

- Many patients needing knee replacement present with retained hardware in femur or tibia.[1-3]
- Conventional intramedullary cutting guides can't be utilized in these patients because of impeding intra- or extramedullary implants, thus necessitating computer-assisted placement of jigs.
- Navigation bypasses the hardware and helps in achieving limb alignment and balance in patients with retained hardware.[4]
- Other possible options for this subset of patients could be:
  - Usage of patient-specific instruments (PSI).
  - Removal of hardware before arthroplasty (partial or complete / staged procedure or single-stage).
  - Handheld navigation.

Pearls

- The patient's history regarding the retained hardware must be considered in detail, particularly ruling out any evidence of *infection*, before planning total knee arthroplasty (TKA).
- Evaluation of the operative site for *planning the skin incision* must be done.
- *Plastic surgery opinion* should be taken for planning the skin incisions or for local flap coverage.

▣ Case Illustrations

- Long-stemmed hip prosthesis.
- United per trochanteric fracture with long proximal femoral nail (PFN) in situ.
- United femoral shaft fracture with locking compression plate (LCP) in situ.
- United femoral shaft fracture with intramedullary nail (IMN) in situ.
- United supracondylar femur fracture with dynamic compression screw (DCS) in situ.
- United femoral shaft fracture with IMN in situ by robotic-assisted surgery.
- United tibial osteotomy with implant in situ.
- Nonunion proximal tibial fracture with implant in situ.
- United proximal tibial diaphyseal fracture with LCP in situ.

Long-Stemmed Hip Prosthesis

- A 60-year-old woman, a known case of rheumatoid arthritis, had undergone bilateral total hip replacement (THR) few years back.
- The patient presented with bilateral knee pain from the last 3 years.
- On examination, the right knee had 10-degree valgus and 10-degree FFD with further flexion up to 120 degrees while the left knee had 20-degree valgus and hyperextension with further flexion up to 130 degrees (**Fig. 8.1**).
- There was no distal neurovascular deficit.
- Kinematic analysis of the left knee showed 16-degree valgus deformity with 6 degrees of hyperextension (**Fig. 8.2**).
- Normal (9.5 mm) distal femur cut (DFC) was taken and verified (**Fig. 8.3**).
- Femoral external rotation was increased to 5 degree taking in account articular cartilage loss from lateral posterior femoral condyle (**Fig. 8.4**).

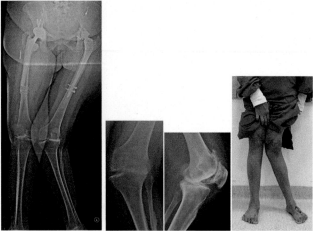

Fig. 8.1 Preoperative radiographs and image of the patient.

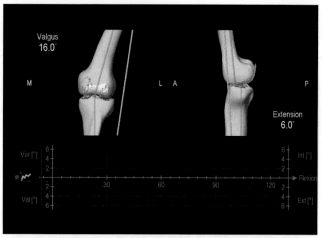

Fig. 8.2 Preoperative limb alignment and kinematics.

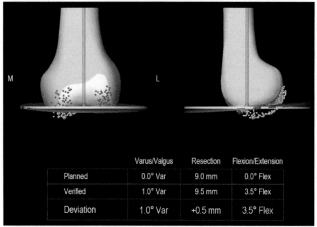

Fig. 8.3 Distal femur cut verification.

	Varus/Valgus	Resection	Flexion/Extension
Planned	0.0° Var	9.0 mm	0.0° Flex
Verified	1.0° Var	9.5 mm	3.5° Flex
Deviation	1.0° Var	+0.5 mm	3.5° Flex

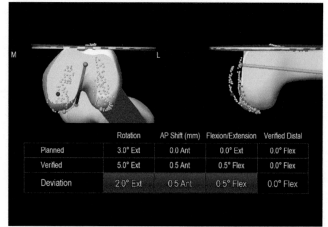

Fig. 8.4 Femoral rotation verification.

	Rotation	AP Shift (mm)	Flexion/Extension	Verified Distal
Planned	3.0° Ext	0.0 Ant	0.0° Ext	0.0° Flex
Verified	5.0° Ext	0.5 Ant	0.5° Flex	0.0° Flex
Deviation	2.0° Ext	0.5 Ant	0.5° Flex	0.0° Flex

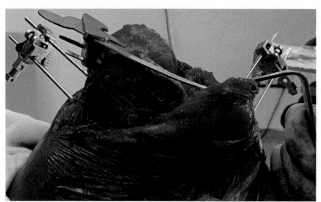

Fig. 8.5 Angel wing to check distal cut thickness.

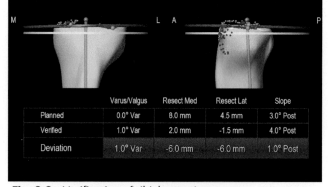

Fig. 8.6 Verification of tibial resection.

	Varus/Valgus	Resect Med	Resect Lat	Slope
Planned	0.0° Var	8.0 mm	4.5 mm	3.0° Post
Verified	1.0° Var	2.0 mm	-1.5 mm	4.0° Post
Deviation	1.0° Var	-6.0 mm	-6.0 mm	1.0° Post

- Angel wing showing minimal resection at lateral femoral condyle (**Fig. 8.5**).
- Conservative proximal tibial cut was taken (**Fig. 8.6**).
- IT band was released to correct the valgus deformity in extension along with popliteus tendon to correct the tight lateral flexion space.

- There was a contained bone defect which was rebuilt with the usage of bone graft and screws.
- Complete correction of deformity in both the sagittal and coronal planes can be seen in postoperative kinematics. (**Fig. 8.7**).
- Bilateral total knee replacement was done utilizing computer navigation (**Fig. 8.8**).

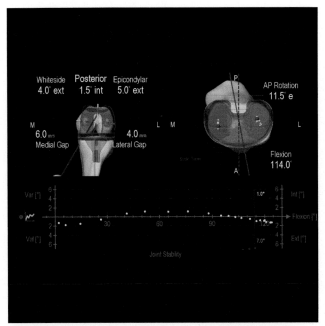

Fig. 8.7 Postoperative limb alignment and kinematics.

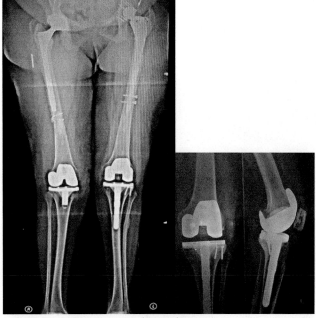

Fig. 8.8 Postoperative radiographs.

- Postoperative radiographs show satisfactory components positioning.
- Bone graft and screws with the intramedullary tibial rod were used for the bone defect in the left knee.

United Per Trochanteric Fracture with Proximal Femoral Nail (PFN) in Situ

- A 70-year-old gentleman presented with bilateral knee pain. There was a history of right proximal femur fracture 10 years back, which was operated with PFN (**Fig. 8.9**).
- There was no evidence of inflammation, swelling, discharge, or scar over the knee joint.
- Preoperative X-rays show bilateral knee arthritis with PFN in situ in the right proximal femur with a united per trochanteric fracture.
- On clinical examination, the right knee had a 15-degree varus deformity with 0 to 120-degree range of motion (ROM).

- The preoperative kinematic graph elicits 13-degree varus deformity with neutral sagittal alignment (**Fig. 8.10**).
- The varus deformity decreased as the knee flexed beyond 90 degrees but didn't correct fully.
- The DFC was decreased as the knee was in hyperextension (**Fig. 8.11**).
- 8.5 mm thickness of bone was resected from the lateral tibial condyle while none was resected from the medial side (**Fig. 8.12**).
- Clinical picture showing proximal tibia cut with minimal bone removed from medial tibial condyle owing to severe varus deformity (**Fig. 8.13**).
- Reduction osteotomy of tibia along with posteromedial soft tissue release were done to correct the deformity.
- The postoperative kinematic graph shows the correction of deformity in both the planes (**Fig. 8.14**).
- The postoperative X-rays show corrected limb alignment with well-positioned knee prosthesis without the need to remove the hardware from the ipsilateral hip. (**Fig. 8.15**).

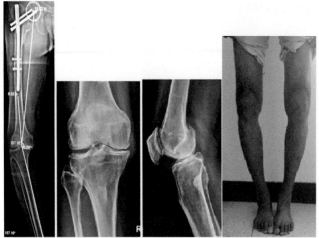

Fig. 8.9 Preoperative radiographs with knee arthritis and proximal femoral nail (PFN) in situ and clinical image of the patient.

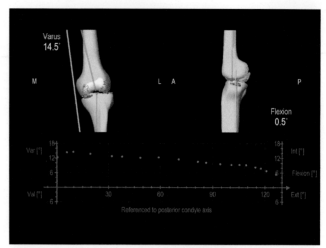

Fig. 8.10 Initial kinematics and deformity.

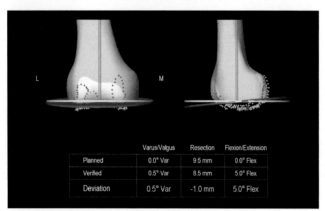

Fig. 8.11 Distal femur resection verification.

	Varus/Valgus	Resection	Flexion/Extension
Planned	0.0° Var	9.5 mm	0.0° Flex
Verified	0.5° Var	8.5 mm	5.0° Flex
Deviation	0.5° Var	-1.0 mm	5.0° Flex

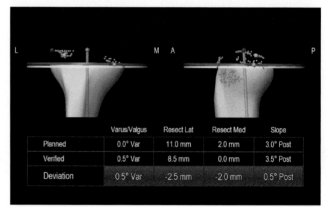

Fig. 8.12 Proximal tibia resection verification.

	Varus/Valgus	Resect Lat	Resect Med	Slope
Planned	0.0° Var	11.0 mm	2.0 mm	3.0° Post
Verified	0.5° Var	8.5 mm	0.0 mm	3.5° Post
Deviation	0.5° Var	-2.5 mm	-2.0 mm	0.5° Post

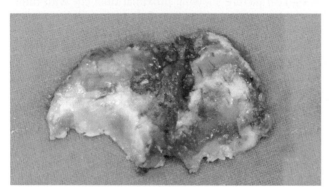

Fig. 8.13 A clinical picture depicting the resected proximal tibia bone with no bone removed from the medial tibial plateau because of the excessive varus deformity.

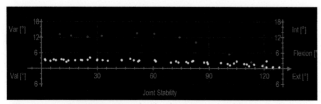

Fig. 8.14 Postoperative limb alignment and kinematics.

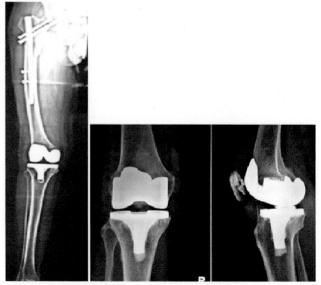

Fig. 8.15 Postoperative radiograph.

United Femoral Shaft Fracture with LCP in Situ

- The patient had a history of comminuted femoral shaft fracture sustained 10 years back, for which open reduction and internal fixation with broad LCP was performed through a lateral approach to the thigh.
- The patient presented with complaints of pain in the knee with difficulty in walking.
- On examination, the patient had 10-degree varus and 15-degree FFD in the left knee with further flexion up to 120 degrees.
- Preoperative radiographs show osteoarthritis of the left knee with united femoral shaft fracture and hardware in situ (**Fig. 8.16** and **Fig. 8.17**).

Pearls

- Computer-assisted surgery (CAS) TKA was done without removing the implant because of the following considerations:
- Technical difficulties anticipated while removing a well-fixed implant inserted a decade back.
- Creation of potential stress risers after implant removal and soft tissue damage associated with the implant removal procedure.

Pitfalls

Patients, who have undergone a previous surgery from a lateral approach, have tight lateral structures such as iliotibial band (ITB) and vastus lateralis. They generally require lateral soft tissue release for patellar maltracking.[5]

- Significant varus (11.5 degree) and flexion deformity (16 degree) was noted on preoperative kinematics (**Fig. 8.18**).
- Extra DFC was taken to correct the flexion deformity (**Fig. 8.19**).
- Due to varus deformity and the associated bony defect in the medial tibial condyle, the proximal tibial cut resulted in minimal bone being resected from the medial condyle as compared to the lateral tibial condyle (**Fig. 8.20** and **Fig. 8.21**).
- Reduction osteotomy of tibia along with posteromedial soft tissue release were done to correct the deformity.
- The navigation graph elicits the postoperative correction of alignment and deformity throughout the complete ROM (**Fig. 8.22**).
- A well-aligned femoral and tibial components without the need for removing previous hardware seen on postoperative radiographs (**Fig. 8.23**).

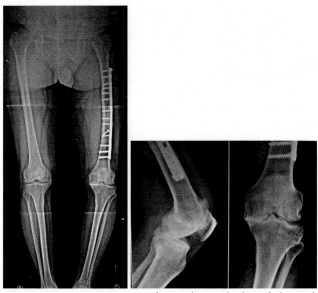

Fig. 8.16 Preoperative radiographs with broad limited contact dynamic compression plate (LC-DCP) in situ.

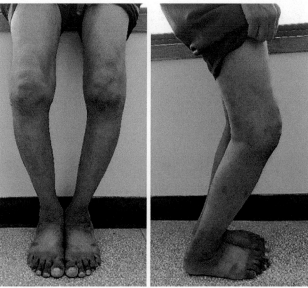

Fig. 8.17 Clinical image of the patient showing varus flexion deformity.

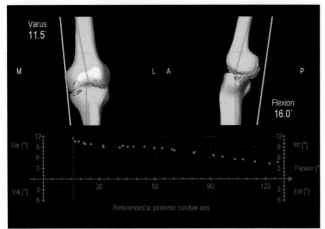

Fig. 8.18 Initial limb alignment and kinematics.

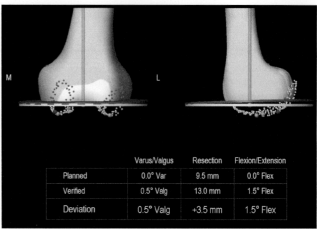

Fig. 8.19 Distal femur resection verification.

	Varus/Valgus	Resection	Flexion/Extension
Planned	0.0° Var	9.5 mm	0.0° Flex
Verified	0.5° Valg	13.0 mm	1.5° Flex
Deviation	0.5° Valg	+3.5 mm	1.5° Flex

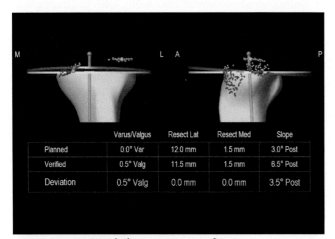

Fig. 8.20 Proximal tibia resection verification.

	Varus/Valgus	Resect Lat	Resect Med	Slope
Planned	0.0° Var	12.0 mm	1.5 mm	3.0° Post
Verified	0.5° Valg	11.5 mm	1.5 mm	6.5° Post
Deviation	0.5° Valg	0.0 mm	0.0 mm	3.5° Post

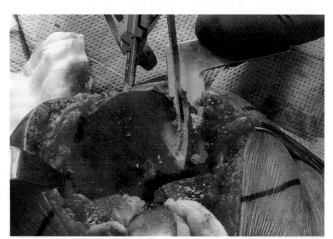

Fig. 8.21 A clinical picture depicting a reduction osteotomy of the tibia being performed to correct the flexion varus deformity.

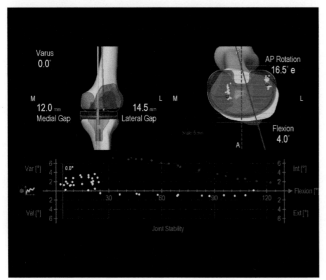

Fig. 8.22 Postoperative limb alignment and corrected kinematics.

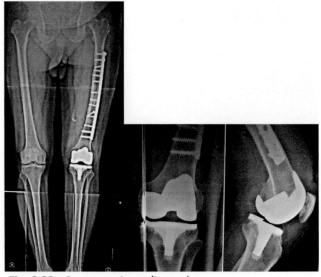

Fig. 8.23 Postoperative radiographs.

United Femoral Shaft Fracture with Intramedullary Nail (IMN) in Situ

- The patient had a history of fracture femur 6 years back, which was fixed with intramedullary nailing (IMN) elsewhere. The distal screws were removed 4 months after the primary procedure due to loosening and back out.
- There was no history of discharge or swelling over the operative site.
- The patient presented with pain in the right knee leading to difficulty in walking for the past 2 years.
- On examination of the right knee joint, there was 15-degree varus and 5-degree FFD with further flexion up to 130 degrees.
- There was osteoarthritis right knee with united femur fracture and IMN in situ in preoperative radiographs. (**Fig. 8.24**).

- Kinematic analysis on navigation shows varus deformity (11.5 degrees) with near neutral sagittal alignment (**Fig. 8.25**).
- On trial, navigation showing residual biplanar deformity (**Fig. 8.26**).
- Correction of tight medial gap (varus) will correct the sagittal deformity (FFD).
- On trial, navigation showed residual varus flexion deformity.
- Downsizing of tibia and removal of posteromedial osteophytes corrects the deformity.
- Tibial component was downsized from size 3 to size 2 (**Fig. 8.27**).
- Residual posteromedial tibial bone was removed with saw after soft tissue releases.
- Postoperative navigation analysis demonstrates complete correction of varus and flexion deformity (**Fig. 8.28**).
- Postoperative radiographs show well-aligned femoral and tibial components, without the need to remove the pre-existing hardware in the femur (**Fig. 8.29**).

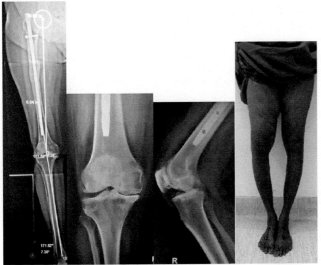

Fig. 8.24 Preoperative radiographs and image of the patient.

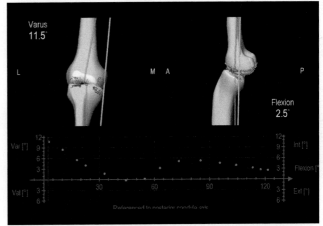

Fig. 8.25 Preoperative kinematics and limb alignment.

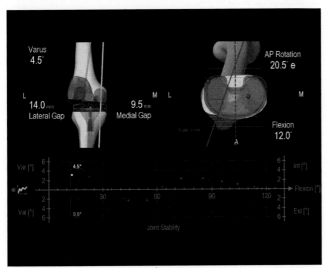

Fig. 8.26 Residual deformity with trials.

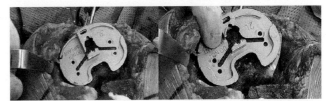

Fig. 8.27 Downsizing tibial tray to relax the tight medial structures.

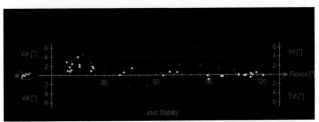

Fig. 8.28 Postoperative limb alignment and corrected kinematics.

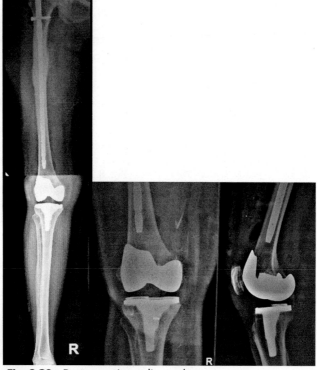

Fig. 8.29 Postoperative radiographs.

United Supracondylar Femur Fracture with Dynamic Compression Screw (DCS) in Situ

- A 70-year-old woman, known case of rheumatoid arthritis, sustained a supracondylar femur fracture 8 years back which was operated with open reduction and internal fixation with DCS.
- On examination, she had less than 5-degree varus, 10-degree FFD with further flexion up to 110 degrees.
- The preoperative radiographs show knee arthritis with osteopenia (**Fig. 8.30**).
- Difficulties were anticipated in the removal of the previous implants, along with the potential to create stress risers after implant removal.
- The surgeon has to be careful of the pre-existing healed skin incisions, to ensure soft tissue viability and to avoid wound-healing complications postoperatively.

- The preoperative clinical image showing healed scar over the anterolateral aspect of the distal left thigh (**Fig. 8.31**).
- The kinematic analysis shows the uncorrectable varus deformity with mild recurvatum (**Fig. 8.32**).
- Details of the DFC verification seen in the navigation values (**Fig. 8.33**).
- The postoperative kinematic analysis shows the correction of the deformities in both the planes (**Fig. 8.34**).
- DCS screw is visible just proximal to the femoral component (**Fig. 8.35**).
- The patella was tracking well with no lift-off.
- Complete correction of the deformity was achieved in both the sagittal and coronal planes without the need to remove the hardware (**Fig. 8.36**).
- Well-aligned tibial and femoral components without the need to remove the pre-existing implant (**Fig. 8.37**).

Pearls

- The distance of the distalmost screw of the implant from the distal femur cut (DFC) was 18 mm, whereas the box cut for the posterior stabilized (PS) knee required 20-mm bony resection. To overcome this, a computer-navigated anterior stabilized TKA was planned.
- The cruciate-retaining (CR) femoral prosthesis was chosen in this case along with anterior stabilized insert.

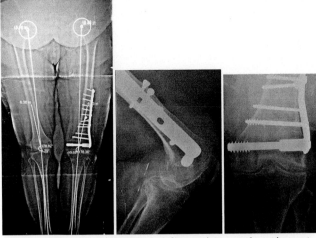

Fig. 8.30 Preoperative radiographs with dynamic compression screw (DCS) in situ.

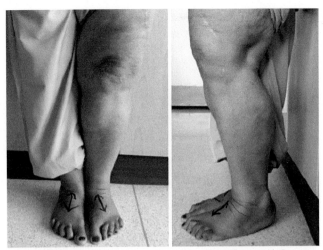

Fig. 8.31 Image of the patient showing flexion deformity and postoperative scar.

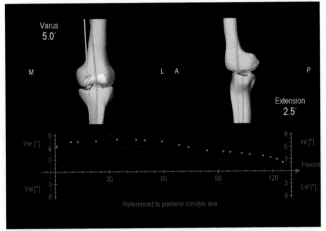

Fig. 8.32 Initial kinematics and limb alignment.

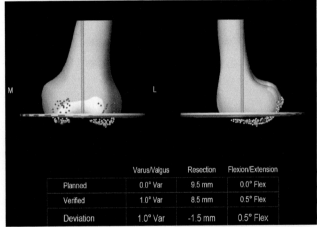

	Varus/Valgus	Resection	Flexion/Extension
Planned	0.0° Var	9.5 mm	0.0° Flex
Verified	1.0° Var	8.5 mm	0.5° Flex
Deviation	1.0° Var	-1.5 mm	0.5° Flex

Fig. 8.33 Distal femur resection verification.

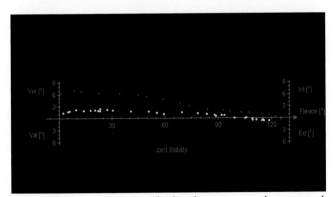

Fig. 8.34 Postoperative limb alignment and corrected kinematics.

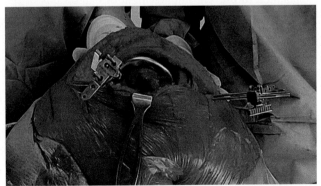

Fig. 8.35 A clinical picture depicting the cruciate-retaining (CR) femoral knee prosthesis with an anterior stabilized insert.

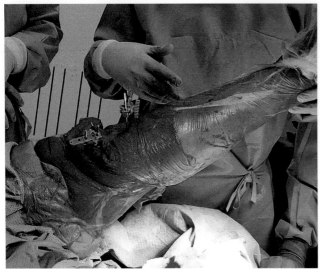

Fig. 8.36 Intraoperative image showing complete correction of deformity.

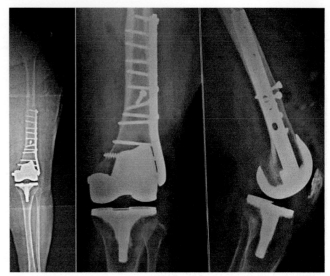

Fig. 8.37 Postoperative radiographs.

United Femoral Shaft Fracture with Intramedullary Nail (IMN) in Situ by Robotic-Assisted Surgery

- The patient sustained femoral shaft fracture 9 years back, for which internal fixation was done with IMN.
- There was complaint of pain in the right knee from the last 1 year.
- On examination of the right knee, there was 10-degree varus deformity, neutral in the sagittal plane, with ROM of 0 to 130 degrees.
- Preoperative radiographs show osteoarthritic right knee with an IMN in situ (**Fig. 8.38**).
- As the distal tip of intramedullary nail would have come in the box of PS knee, a cruciate retaining knee was planned to prevent impingement of nail on box of the knee.

Pearls

- Robotics provides additional information about the soft tissue behavior along with quantifying the coronal and sagittal plane deformities.
- These cases require precise planning to be done to attain the desired correction with limited scope for additional cuts.
- In robotics, the bony cuts are taken by a robotic burr, so the surgeon has better control over the depth of bony resection than an oscillating saw.

- Initial planning shows deformity and implant size predicted by robotics system (**Fig. 8.39**).
- Distal femur was burred and verified using verification probe to check alignment (**Fig. 8.40**).
- Similarly, proximal tibia is burred instead of resection and verified with verification probe (**Fig. 8.41**).
- Postoperative gap assessment shows 1 to 2 mm of gap opening throughout ROM (**Fig. 8.42**).
- Final case report showing alignment and ligament balance (**Fig. 8.43**).
- Well-aligned tibial and femoral components without the need for removing the femoral nail seen in postoperative radiographs (**Fig. 8.44**).

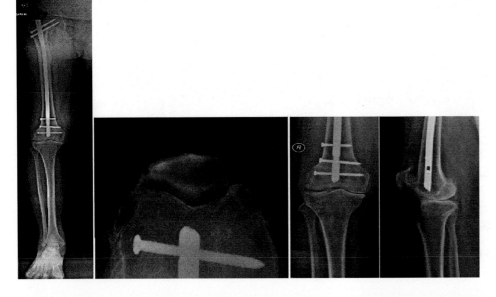

Fig. 8.38 Preoperative radiographs.

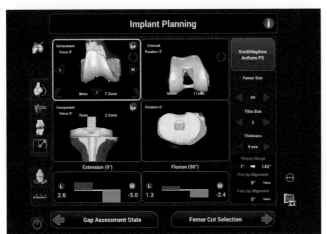

Fig. 8.39 Robotic screen showing initial implant planning.

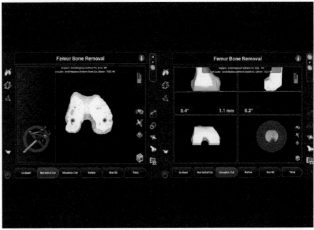

Fig. 8.40 Initial distal femur burr and cut verification.

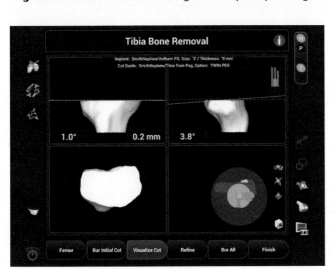

Fig. 8.41 Proximal tibia burr verification.

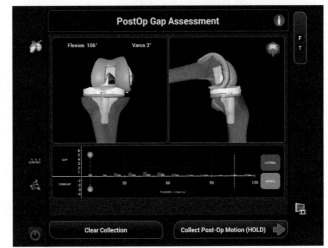

Fig. 8.42 Postoperative gap assessment.

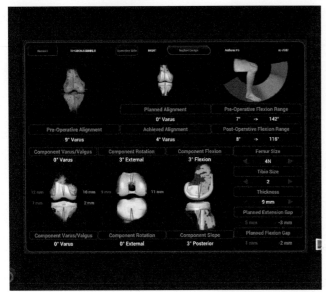

Fig. 8.43 Final report of the case.

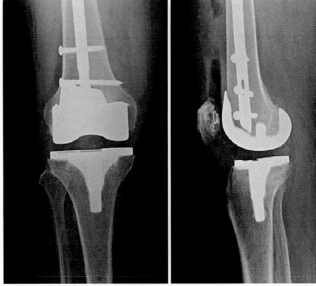

Fig. 8.44 Postoperative radiographs.

United Tibial Osteotomy with Implant in Situ

- A 55-year-old woman presented with complain of pain in left knee and difficulty in walking.
- She had a history of left medial open-wedge osteotomy performed 10 years back.
- On examination, the ROM of the left knee joint was 10 to 120 degrees, with a varus deformity of 10 degrees.
- Implants were removed with extended medial parapatellar incision.
- The tibial navigation pins were placed distally in the diaphyseal part of the tibia.
- Preoperative radiographs show medial compartment arthritis with a paradoxical valgus joint line (medial plateau is higher than the lateral plateau in spite of medial compartment arthritis) (**Fig. 8.45**),
- Upward tibial slope is also seen on the lateral view which is a common finding post HTO.

- Navigation screen showing mild varus (3.5 degree) with recurvatum deformity (4.5 degree) (**Fig. 8.46**).
- Postosteotomy arthritis usually presents with recurvatum deformity because of reversal of tibial slope.
- Distal femur resection was decreased by 1 to 1.5 mm to keep knee in 5 to 7 degrees of flexion postoperatively (**Fig. 8.47**).
- Minimal tibial resection was done to balance the knee (**Fig. 8.48**).
- It is advisable to keep slope between 3 and 5 degrees to balance loose flexion gap.
- Postoperative kinematics showing well-balanced knee throughout ROM (**Fig. 8.49**).
- Knee was kept in 7 degrees of residual flexion to prevent recurrence of recurvatum deformity.
- The postoperative radiographs have well-aligned knee components after removal of the tibial implant (**Fig. 8.50**).

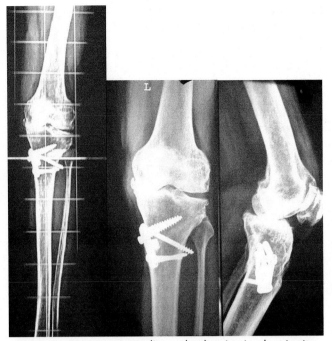

Fig. 8.45 Preoperative radiographs showing implant in situ.

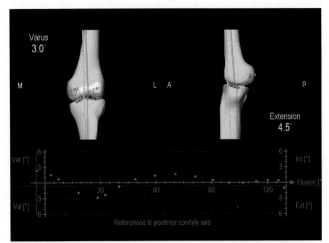

Fig. 8.46 Preoperative limb alignment and kinematics.

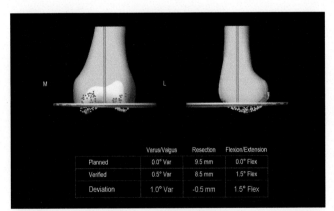

Fig. 8.47 Distal femur cut verification.

	Varus/Valgus	Resection	Flexion/Extension
Planned	0.0° Var	9.5 mm	0.0° Flex
Verified	0.5° Var	8.5 mm	1.5° Flex
Deviation	1.0° Var	-0.5 mm	1.5° Flex

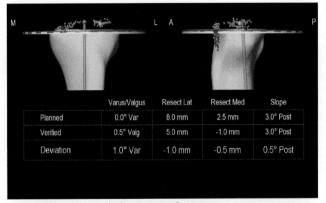

Fig. 8.48 Proximal tibia cut verification.

	Varus/Valgus	Resect Lat	Resect Med	Slope
Planned	0.0° Var	8.0 mm	2.5 mm	3.0° Post
Verified	0.5° Valg	5.0 mm	-1.0 mm	3.0° Post
Deviation	1.0° Var	-1.0 mm	-0.5 mm	0.5° Post

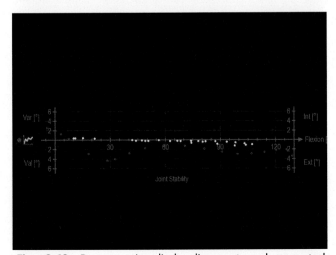

Fig. 8.49 Postoperative limb alignment and corrected kinematics.

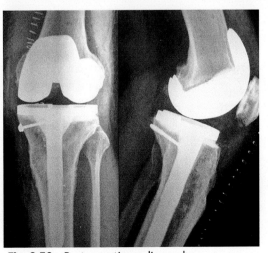

Fig. 8.50 Postoperative radiographs.

Nonunion Proximal Tibial Fracture with Implant in Situ

- The patient had a history of proximal tibia fracture, sustained 2 years back, which was operated and fixed with medial plate and screws elsewhere.
- There was no history of discharge or swelling over the operative site.

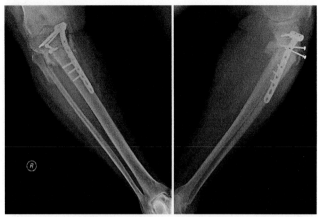

Fig. 8.51 Preoperative radiographs showing implant in situ.

- Blood markers ESR and CRP were within normal limits.
- The patient presented with pain in the right knee leading to difficulty in walking for the past 1 year.
- On examination of the joint, there was mild varus and severe flexion deformity with ROM of 20 to 90 degrees.
- Posttraumatic right knee arthritis and nonunion of proximal tibia with implants in situ seen on preoperative radiographs (**Fig. 8.51**).
- Preoperative image of the knee showing flexion deformity and screw impingement (**Fig. 8.52**).
- Preoperative kinematics analysis showed severe flexion deformity of 16 degrees and 5 degrees of varus (**Fig. 8.53**).
- ROM was restricted to 100 degrees after adhesiolysis and osteophyte removal.
- Additional distal femur cut with mild posteromedial soft tissue release was done to correct the deformity.
- Complete correction of flexion and varus deformity with increased ROM to 120 degrees and beyond on postoperative kinematics analysis. (**Fig. 8.54**).
- There were well-fixed implants with long stem to bypass fracture site in postoperative radiographs. (**Fig. 8.55**).
- A medial plate was added to provide rotational support.

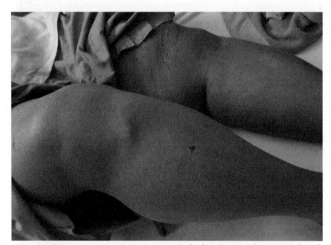

Fig. 8.52 Preoperative image of the knee showing fixed flexion deformity.

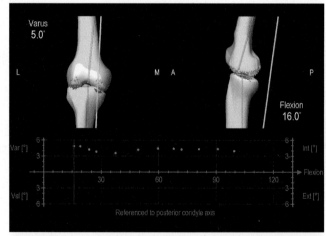

Fig. 8.53 Preoperative limb alignment and kinematics.

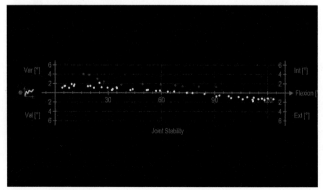

Fig. 8.54 Postoperative limb alignment and corrected kinematics.

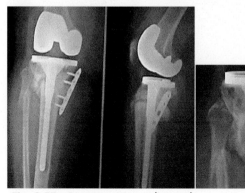

Fig. 8.55 Postoperative radiographs.

United Proximal Tibial Diaphyseal Fracture with LCP in Situ

- A 74-year-old obese gentleman with a BMI of 42.6 kg/m² and a previous history of 20-year-old united proximal tibial diaphyseal fracture with LCP in situ, presented with left knee pain.
- On examination, the ROM of the left knee joint was 0 to 110 degrees, with a varus deformity.
- Preoperative radiographs show subluxed left knee with united proximal tibial diaphyseal fracture and an implant in situ (**Fig. 8.56**).
- Only the proximal screws were removed to accommodate tibial prosthesis.
- The plate was not removed as it would have required a longer incision and created stress riser which could have predisposed to stress fracture.
- The tibial navigation pins were placed distally in the diaphyseal part of the tibia.

- The navigation graph demonstrated a biplanar deformity of varus (11 degrees) with hyperextension (2 degrees) (**Fig. 8.57**).
- Since there is varus hyperextension deformity, a conservative DFC was taken to manage loose extension gap (**Fig. 8.58**).
- 8-mm proximal tibia cut with a 4-degree posterior slope was planned (**Fig. 8.59**).
- Posteromedial soft tissues were released with removal of medial tibial osteophytes to correct the varus deformity.
- A residual 6-mm medial tibial condyle defect was managed with a screw.
- Intraoperative image showing medial tibial condyle defect, managed with a screw (**Fig. 8.60**).
- Complete correction of biplanar deformity seen on postoperative kinematic graph (**Fig. 8.61**).
- Well-aligned and well-balanced knee seen on postoperative radiographs. The plate is still in situ and tibial implant was inserted by removing only proximal two screws (**Fig. 8.62**).

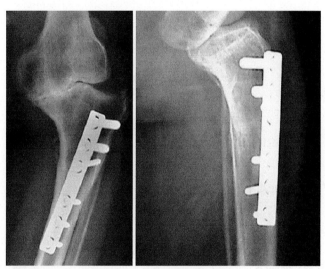

Fig. 8.56 Preoperative radiographs.

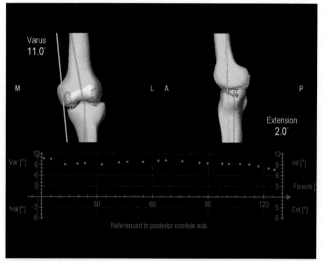

Fig. 8.57 Preoperative limb alignment and kinematics.

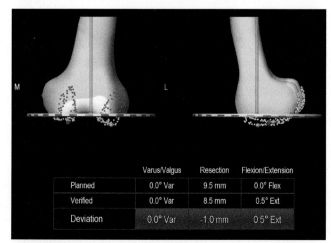

Fig. 8.58 Distal femur cut verification.

	Varus/Valgus	Resection	Flexion/Extension
Planned	0.0° Var	9.5 mm	0.0° Flex
Verified	0.0° Var	8.5 mm	0.5° Ext
Deviation	0.0° Var	-1.0 mm	0.5° Ext

Fig. 8.59 Proximal tibia cut verification.

	Varus/Valgus	Resect Lat	Resect Med	Slope
Planned	0.0° Var	9.0 mm	2.0 mm	3.0° Post
Verified	0.0° Var	7.5 mm	0.5 mm	4.0° Post
Deviation	0.0° Var	-1.5 mm	-1.5 mm	1.0° Post

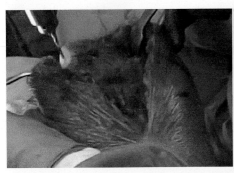
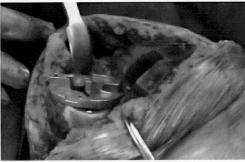

Fig. 8.60 Screw for medial tibial condyle defect.

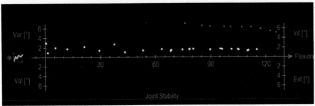

Fig. 8.61 Postoperative limb alignment and corrected kinematics.

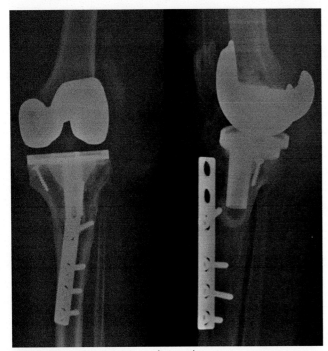

Fig. 8.62 Postoperative radiographs.

Points to Remember

- The surgeon has to rule out infection and give due consideration to potential hardware complications before planning a TKA in patients with retained hardware around the knee joint.[5]
- Staged procedures are recommended for suspected infections or the management of a difficult wound.[6]
- The partial removal of previous hardware is a reasonable surgical option, provided the retained hardware does not interfere with bony preparation or prosthesis positioning.[7]

- The surgeon has to be careful of the skin incisions, to ensure soft tissue viability and to avoid healing complications postoperatively.
- Incision for TKA should be planned meticulously as posttraumatic knees usually have increased scar tissue and contractures.
- A thorough clinical and radiological evaluation of the previous fracture site is desirable to ascertain the union status. Pain in the knee could be originating due to failure of complete union of the previous fracture site.
- Computer navigation helps in executing TKA in patients with retained hardware eliminating the need to remove implants, additional incision, and soft tissue trauma.

References

1. Tigani D, Masetti G, Sabbioni G, Ben Ayad R, Filanti M, Fosco M. Computer-assisted surgery as indication of choice: total knee arthroplasty in case of retained hardware or extra-articular deformity. Int Orthop 2012;36(7):1379–1385

2. Hernandez-Vaquero D, Suarez-Vazquez A, Iglesias-Fernandez S. Computer-assisted navigation in total knee arthroplasty without femoral hardware removal. Acta Chir Orthop Traumatol Cech 2012;79(4):331–24

3. Lin SY, Chen CH, Huang PJ, Fu YC, Huang HT. Computer-navigated minimally invasive total knee arthroplasty for patients with retained implants in the femur. Kaohsiung J Med Sci 2014;30(8):415–421

4. Hamada D, Egawa H, Goto T, et al. Navigation-assisted total knee arthroplasty for osteoarthritis with extra-articular femoral deformity and/or retained hardware. Case Rep Orthop 2013;2013:174384

5. Varacallo M, Johanson NA. Total knee Arthroplasty (TKA) techniques. Treasure Island (FL): StatPearls Publishing LLC; 2018. https://www.ncbi.nlm.nih.gov/books/NBK499896/

6. Shaikh AA, Ha CW, Park YG, Park YB. Two-stage approach to primary TKA in infected arthritic knees using intraoperatively molded articulating cement spacers. Clin Orthop Relat Res 2014;472(7):2201–2207

7. Manrique J, Rasouli MR, Restrepo C, et al. Total knee arthroplasty in patients with retention of prior hardware material: what is the outcome? Arch Bone Jt Surg 2018;6(1):23–26

Computer-Navigated TKR in Special Situations

9

Anoop Jhurani and Piyush Agarwal

Introduction

- Computer navigation has added advantage in total knee arthroplasty (TKA) for systemic conditions like ankylosing spondylitis, rheumatoid arthritis, obesity, foot deformities, etc.
- These systemic diseases have deformities and arthritis of other joints like spine and hips which can influence knee alignment and function post-TKA.
- Knee deformities in these conditions can be severe and profound along with soft tissue abnormalities.
- Conventional TKA can lead to malalignment and imbalance because of associated joint and bony anomalies.
- This chapter focuses on use of computer navigation and its advantages in the following conditions:
  - Morbid obesity.
  - Rheumatoid arthritis.
  - Ankylosing spondylitis.
  - Alkaptonuria.
  - Diffuse idiopathic skeletal hyperostosis (DISH).
  - Foot deformity.
  - Miscellaneous.

Morbid Obesity

- Obesity is an independent risk factor for early arthritis and may require surgical intervention at a younger age.[1]
- WHO has prescribed standard guidelines for defining the severity of obesity, as per the body mass index (BMI)[2]:
  - 18.5 to 25 kg/m² = Normal.
  - 25 to 30 kg/m² = Overweight.
  - 30 to 35 kg/m² = Obese.
  - 35 to 40 kg/m² ⁼ Severe obesity.
  - 40 to 50 kg/m² = Morbid obesity.
  - >50 kg/m² = Super obese.

- The majority of obese patients have associated medical comorbidities like diabetes mellitus, cardiovascular disease, renal insufficiency, obstructive sleep apnea, or pulmonary disease. A multidisciplinary team approach is required to optimize them before surgery.
- Obese patients undergoing TKA have an increased risk of perioperative complications as compared to the non-obese ones.[3]
- Morbidly obese patients have a higher incidence of postoperative complications such as infection, periprosthetic fractures, wound dehiscence, and anterior knee pain.[3]
- Super obese patients have the highest risk of complications and the worst functional outcomes as compared to other categories of obese patients.
- Literature reports conflicting results regarding the prosthesis survival in obese individuals. While some studies show an insignificant change in survivorship of the implants in an obese patient, others suggest an increased incidence of aseptic loosening causing early failure.[4,5]
- A healthy weight loss before undergoing arthroplasty is considered desirable. However, if extreme measures are taken to achieve the weight loss before surgery, the patient's healing potential may be compromised, affecting their ability to handle the physiological stress of the procedure.[6]
- Morbidly obese patients who undergo TKA report improved knee scores, greater relief in pain, and higher satisfaction levels postoperatively as compared to non-obese individuals.[7]
- The advantages of using computer navigation for performing TKA in an obese patient are:
  - Accurate assessment of the deformity which may be difficult through conventional methods because of fat accumulation around bony landmarks.
  - Greater precision in planning bony cuts and soft tissue releases.

During conventional TKA, there is an increased chance of varus tibial cut due to displacement of the extramedullary tibial jig by the subcutaneous fat.[8] The resulting malpositioned tibial component has a greater probability of aseptic loosening and early prosthesis failure because of excessive weight and osteoporosis.[9] Navigation helps in minimizing this risk by ensuring appropriate prosthesis positioning.

Case Illustration

- A 65-year-old woman presented with bilateral knee pain and restricted activities of daily living (ADL).
- Patient also had diabetes mellitus, hypertension, hypothyroidism and metabolic syndrome.
- Bilateral knee range of motion (ROM) was 0 to 90 degrees with severe varus deformity (**Fig. 9.1**).
- Patient's weight was 110 kg with a height of 154 cm. The BMI was 46.4 kg/m², thus categorizing the patient as morbidly obese.
- Preoperative radiographs show varus alignment, tricompartmental osteoarthritis with lateral subluxation of the left knee joint.
- Soft tissue shadows suggest fat folds due to morbid obesity.

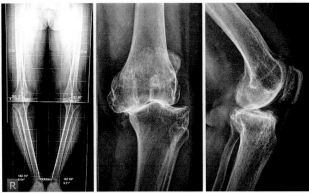

Fig. 9.1 Preoperative radiographs.

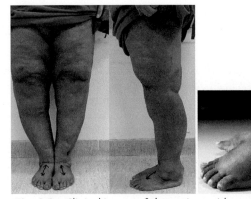

Fig. 9.2 Clinical image of the patient with swelling over feet and ankle.

- The clinical pictures depict the excessive subcutaneous fat in a morbidly obese patient, masking the bony landmarks, especially around the ankle joint. This renders it challenging to accurately locate the bony points during the registration process (**Fig. 9.2**).

Preoperative Preparation

- It is advisable to keep the patients informed of the increased surgical complication rate with higher BMI. This helps to set realistic expectations of surgical outcomes.
- Obese patients have an increased incidence of anterior knee pain after TKA and should be counseled accordingly.[1]
- Preoperative weight loss, including bariatric surgery, is encouraged if deemed necessary. There is no specific cutoff of BMI for advising bariatric surgery before joint replacement.

Intraoperative Preparation

- Tourniquet usage:
  - A wider, low-pressure tourniquet should be utilized to prevent any iatrogenic neurovascular injury.
  - It should be applied as proximally as possible on the thigh to allow for wide surgical exposure.
  - The authors use the tourniquet more as a tool to pull thigh fat distally and to help in draping (**Fig. 9.3**).
- Surgical approach and exposure:
  - Wide exposure of the knee joint may be required.
  - The authors use a midline approach with medial parapatellar arthrotomy in all the cases.
  - Eversion of the patella can be challenging in obese patients because of the fat pad and patella baja associated with the majority of the cases.
  - Navigation pins need to be inserted proximally in the femur and distally in the tibia to prevent compression of the soft tissues intraoperatively.
- Single-layer iodinated draping is recommended over the ankle, to facilitate palpation and correct registration.

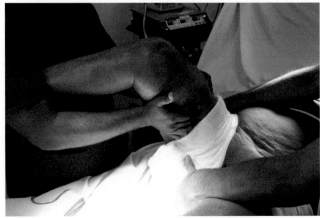

Fig. 9.3 Tourniquet application over fatty thigh.

- In obese patients, pins should be placed proximally in the femur, as increased bulk of the thigh makes it difficult to elevate the femur in flexion (**Fig. 9.4**).
- The preoperative navigation graph shows severe varus deformity (20 degrees) with recurvatum (1.5 degrees) (**Fig. 9.5**).
- A conservative distal femur cut should be taken in obese patients as most of them have ligament laxity and occult recurvatum (**Fig. 9.6** and **Fig. 9.7**).

- The excessive thigh fat makes it difficult to appreciate the sagittal deformity clinically.
- The authors aim to keep the knee in 5 to 7 degrees of flexion postoperatively to prevent recurrence of recurvatum.
- A conservative tibial cut is taken in obese patients as soft tissues are lax and gaps are loose (**Fig. 9.8** and **Fig. 9.9**).

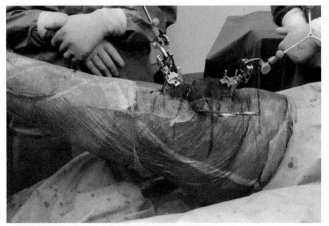

Fig. 9.4 Bulky thigh with navigation arrays.

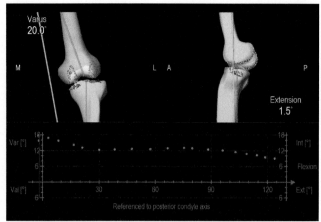

Fig. 9.5 Initial limb alignment and kinematics.

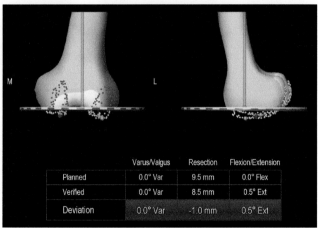

	Varus/Valgus	Resection	Flexion/Extension
Planned	0.0° Var	9.5 mm	0.0° Flex
Verified	0.0° Var	8.5 mm	0.5° Ext
Deviation	0.0° Var	-1.0 mm	0.5° Ext

Fig. 9.6 Distal femur resection verification.

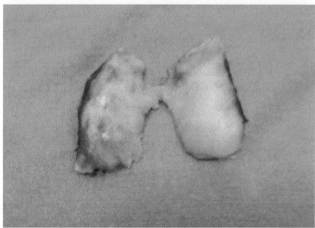

Fig. 9.7 Distal femur cut.

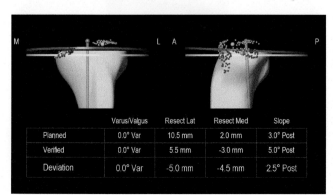

	Varus/Valgus	Resect Lat	Resect Med	Slope
Planned	0.0° Var	10.5 mm	2.0 mm	3.0° Post
Verified	0.0° Var	5.5 mm	-3.0 mm	5.0° Post
Deviation	0.0° Var	-5.0 mm	-4.5 mm	2.5° Post

Fig. 9.8 Proximal tibia cut verification.

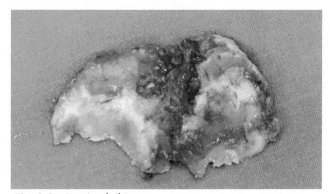

Fig. 9.9 Proximal tibia cut.

- Navigation assists in determining accurate positioning of an extramedullary tibial cutting jig, thus facilitating an accurate tibial cut.
- A residual 6 degrees of flexion as planned previously, with complete correction of the coronal plane deformity throughout the range of motion can be seen on postoperative navigation screen (**Fig. 9.10**).
- The postoperative radiographs depicted well-aligned components (**Fig. 9.11**).
- Knees should be kept in 2 to 3 degrees varus to prevent the thighs from rubbing each other. Neutral or valgus alignment can make it difficult for the patient to walk because of attrition of thigh fat (**Fig. 9.12**).
- Prosthesis considerations:
  - The authors recommend using an additional short cemented stem in tibia for load sharing and to decrease stress on the tibial baseplate.
  - The authors advocate resurfacing the patella in all the cases, as obese patients have higher incidence of postoperative anterior knee pain.
- Meticulous soft tissue handling:
  - The medial collateral ligament (MCL) is at a greater risk of injury in an obese patient and must be protected at all times during the procedure.

- Proper balancing of the knee is critical. The excessive weight of the lower limb may give a false sense of stability. Actual instability may be elicited by lifting the femur.
- Meticulous closure should be performed in layers, as obese patients have a higher risk of wound complications postoperatively.

Postoperatively

- The surgical site should be closely monitored as there is an increased risk of postoperative infection and fat necrosis among obese patients.[10]
- Patients should be encouraged to perform ankle pump exercises to prevent DVT and to frequently change position in bed to prevent pressure sores.
- The surgeon should encourage an early range of motion and active physiotherapy in these patients on ward rounds.
- Patients need to be counseled regarding anticipated initial pain, slow recovery, and decreased range of motion. They should be continuously motivated to adhere to the physiotherapy program.

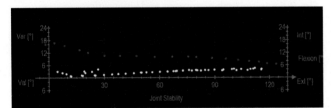

Fig. 9.10 Final limb alignment and kinematics.

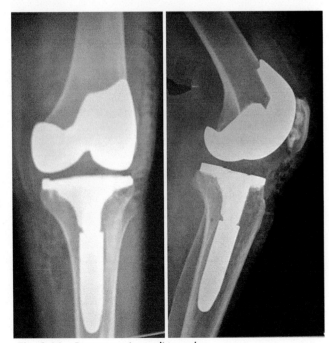

Fig. 9.11 Postoperative radiographs.

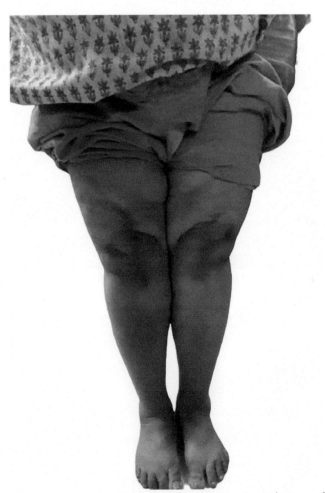

Fig. 9.12 Obese patient should be kept in 2 to 3 degrees of overall mechanical varus.

- Medial femoral condyle is prepared with a burr in exposure control mode (**Fig. 10.23**).
- 3D model of femur and tibia shows removed bone (**Fig. 10.24**).

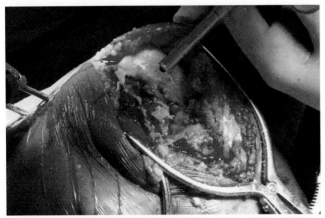

Fig. 10.23 Femur burring.

- Peg holes for femur component are prepared with spherical or cylindrical burr in speed control speed mode (**Fig. 10.25** and **Fig. 10.26**).
- A clinical picture showing the prosthesis trial components in situ (**Fig. 10.27**).
- Postoperative ROM shows final alignment of 3-degree varus and 7-degree flexion (**Fig. 10.28**).
- Postoperative long leg radiograph shows overall mechanical alignment in 2 to 3 degrees of varus which is the goal in UKA (**Fig. 10.29**).
- The AP radiograph shows well-aligned femur component on tibial component without overhang of either of the parts.
- The lateral X-ray shows correct sizing of the femur component with no overhang beyond tidemark point. The tibial slope is also restored to the preoperative native slope.

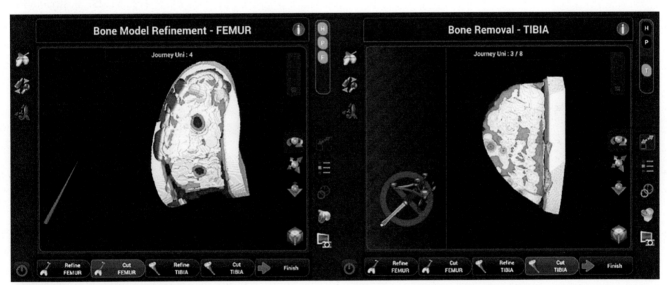

Fig. 10.24 3D model postburring.

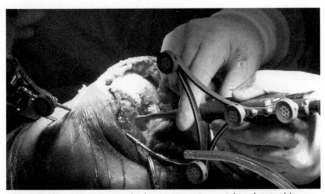

Fig. 10.25 Femur peg hole preparation with spherical burr.

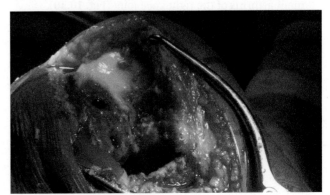

Fig. 10.26 Femur peg holes.

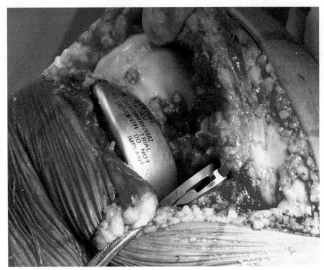

Fig. 10.27 Trial components.

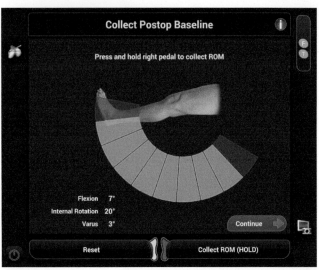

Fig. 10.28 Postoperative range of motion (ROM) and final alignment.

Fig. 10.29 Postoperative radiographs.

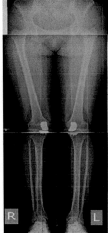
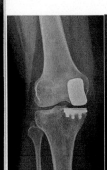
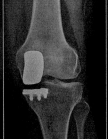
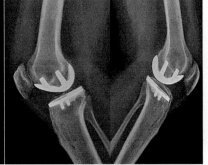

Case 2

- The preoperative radiographs show medial compartment arthritis of the right knee joint (**Fig. 10.30**).
- Intraoperatively, it was confirmed that the arthritic changes are restricted to the medial compartment of knee and medial facet of patella (**Fig. 10.31**).

Pearls

- Patellofemoral arthritis should be restricted to the medial facet of patella.
- If the changes extend to the lateral facet of patella or the lateral femoral condyle, then it is a contraindication for partial knee replacement.

- The preoperative kinematics analysis elicit a tight flexion gap beyond 30-degree range of movement (orange dotted line below the midline) (**Fig. 10.32**)

- Gap balancing (orange dotted line brought above the midline which represents gap opening of 1-2mm throughout ROM) done by following component adjustments (**Fig. 10.33**):
  - The femoral component brought superiorly and downsized to increase the flexion gap.
  - Resection of femoral component was planned in 1-degree varus.
  - Planning such knees with the femoral component in 0.5 to 1 degree of varus helps in achieving a neutral alignment after burring the bone.
  - The depth of the tibial cut was reduced to 4 mm to balance the gaps.
  - The residual varus was reduced to 3 degrees.
- Picture showing automatic stopping of the burring activity by retraction of burr when the burr moved accidentally over the lateral condyle which lay outside the resection plan (**Fig. 10.34**).
- While using speed control mode during tibial burring, ACL footprint should be protected from damage (**Fig. 10.35**).

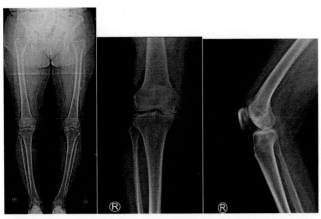

Fig. 10.30 Preoperative radiographs.

- Spacer block is used to check flexion extension gaps before the trails are inserted (**Fig. 10.36**).
- The postoperative stressed gap assessment shows joint opening of 1 to 2 mm during the entire ROM (**Fig. 10.37**).
- The knee had a residual flexion deformity of 7 degrees with 3-degree residual varus alignment. Authors prefer to keep in 5- to 7-degree flexion which comes to neutral when patient bears weight.
- Holes are drilled with 2-mm K-wire in femur and tibia for improved cement penetration (**Fig. 10.38**).
- The postoperative radiographs show a well-balanced knee with satisfactory prosthesis positioning (**Fig. 10.39**).
- The patient was able to comfortably sit cross-legged postoperatively.

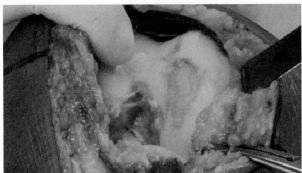
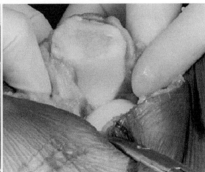

Fig. 10.31 Medial condyle arthritis.

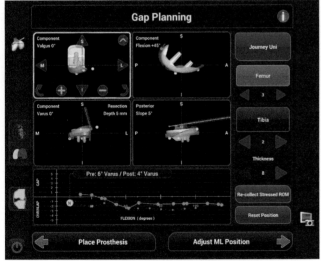

Fig. 10.32 Initial planning and gap balance.

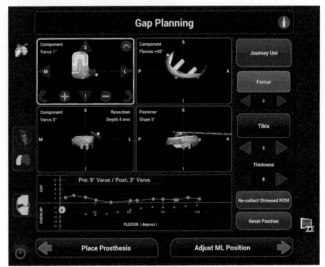

Fig. 10.33 Post planning and gap balance.

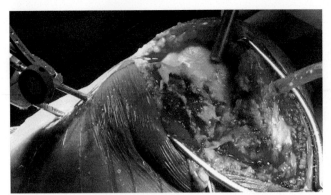

Fig. 10.34 Femur burring stops at lateral condyle.

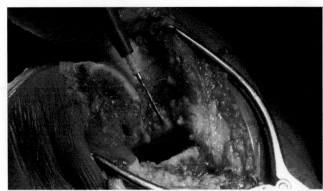

Fig. 10.35 Preserved anterior cruciate ligament (ACL) footprint.

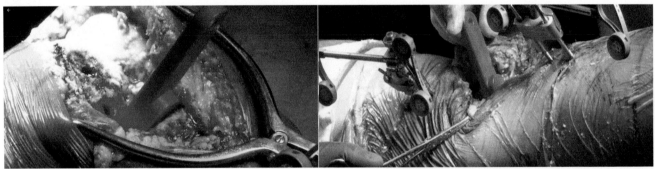

Fig. 10.36 Spacer block to check adequate gap and balance in flexion and extension.

Postop Stressed Gap Assessment

Manufacturer/Design	SmithNephew / Journey Uni
Femur Size	2
Tibia Size/Thickness	2 / 8
Pre-Operative Alignment	6° Varus
Planned Alignment	5° Varus

Flexion 7°
Internal Rotation 1°
Varus 3°

Reset | Release to Stop

Fig. 10.37 Postoperative gap assessment.

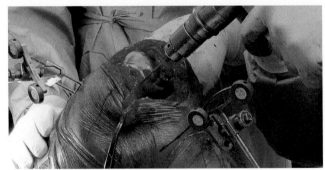

Fig. 10.38 K-wire for drill holes.

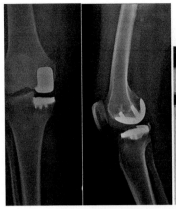
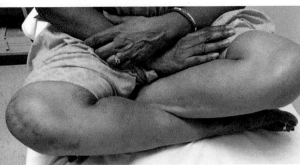

Fig. 10.39 Postoperative radiographs and range of motion (ROM) at 6 months.

Case 3

- The preoperative radiographs show medial compartment arthritis with opening on valgus stress view (**Fig. 10.40** to **Fig. 10.42**).
- The preoperative kinematics analysis of the patient show loose extension and flexion gaps (**Fig. 10.43**).
- Gap planning was done by the following component adjustments (**Fig. 10.44**):
  - The femur component was brought distally and inferiorly to tighten the extension and flexion gaps.
  - Upsizing of the femoral component was not done since there was significant overhanging with size 5.
  - The femoral component was kept in 1-degree varus to compensate for the tight medial gap.
  - The tibial component size was increased to cover the exposed bone.
  - Final expected alignment was in 1-degree varus.
- The postoperative range of movement analysis shows residual 6-degree flexion with 3-degree varus (**Fig. 10.45**).

- A well-balanced knee with 1 to 2 mm opening in the entire ROM seen on postoperative gap assessment (**Fig. 10.46**).
- Tibia is cemented first followed by femur (**Fig. 10.47**). The femoral component goes in 45 degree of flexion as the peg holes are in the same plane as the sagittal axis of femur.

Pearls

Minimal cement should be used posteriorly on the femur and tibial component to prevent extrusion of the cement in the posterior capsule which may be difficult to remove.

- Well-aligned UKA components seen on postoperative radiographs (**Fig. 10.48**).

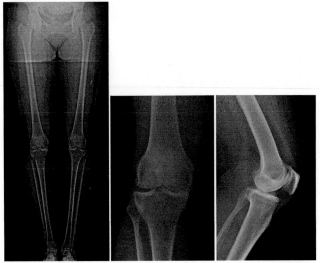

Fig. 10.40 Preoperative radiographs.

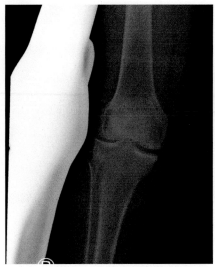

Fig. 10.41 Valgus stress view.

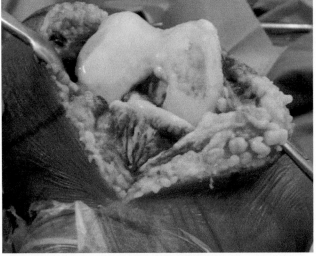

Fig. 10.42 Medial condyle osteoarthritis.

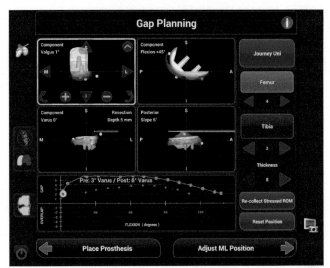

Fig. 10.43 Initial planning and gap balance.

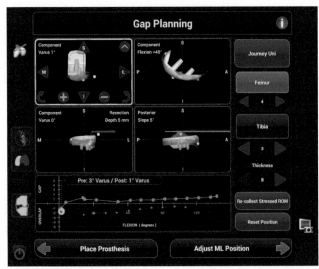

Fig. 10.44 Post planning and gap balance.

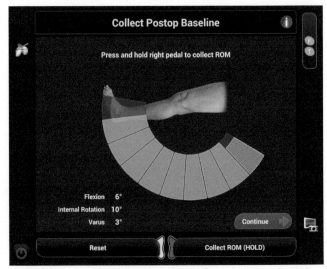

Fig. 10.45 Postoperative baseline range of motion (ROM).

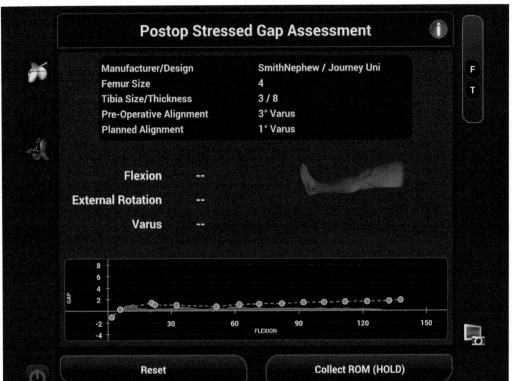

Fig. 10.46 Postoperative stress gap assessment.

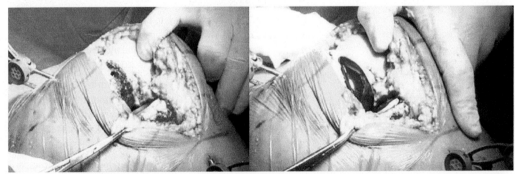

Fig. 10.47 Implant cementation.

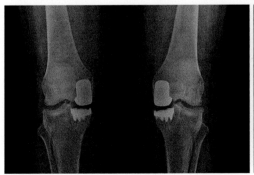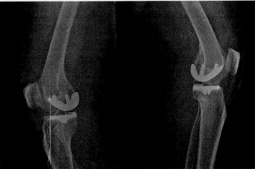

Fig. 10.48 Postoperative radiographs.

Points to Remember

- A medial UKA is indicated if there is full thickness cartilage loss of medial tibiofemoral compartment.
- The varus and fixed flexion deformity should not be more than 10 degrees in the respective planes.
- ACL should be intact and the joint should open on valgus stress X-ray indicating that the MCL has no permanent contracture.
- Patellar arthritic changes should be restricted to medial facet of patella.
- Robotics gives accurate assessment of deformity and helps in gap balancing.
- Most planning can be done by moving the femur component.
- The tibial resection is always 4 to 5mm with 5 to 7 degree slope.
- The femur component is moved distally if the extension gap is loose or proximally if the extension gap is tight.
- The femur component can also be moved superiorly or inferiorly based on tightness or laxity of flexion space.
- Robotics has shown to decrease the complications on tibial side because of minimal tibial bone resection and avoidance of tibial pins for jig placement.

References

1. Ackroyd CE. Medial compartment arthroplasty of the knee. J Bone Joint Surg Br 2003;85(7):937–942

2. Siman H, Kamath AF, Carrillo N, Harmsen WS, Pagnano MW, Sierra RJ. Unicompartmental knee arthroplasty vs total knee arthroplasty for medial compartment arthritis in patients older than 75 years: comparable reoperation, revision, and complication rates. J Arthroplasty 2017;32(6):1792–1797

3. Arirachakaran A, Choowit P, Putananon C, Muangsiri S, Kongtharvonskul J. Is unicompartmental knee arthroplasty (UKA) superior to total knee arthroplasty (TKA)? A systematic review and meta-analysis of randomized controlled trial. Eur J Orthop Surg Traumatol 2015;25(5):799–806

4. Murray DW, Liddle AD, Judge A, Pandit H. Bias and unicompartmental knee arthroplasty. Bone Joint J 2017;99-B(1):12–15

5. Kayani B, Haddad FS. Robotic unicompartmental knee arthroplasty: Current challenges and future perspectives. Bone Joint Res 2019;8(6):228–231

6. Herry Y, Batailler C, Lording T, Servien E, Neyret P, Lustig S. Improved joint-line restitution in unicompartmental knee arthroplasty using a robotic-assisted surgical technique. Int Orthop 2017;41(11):2265–2271

7. Plate JF, Mofidi A, Mannava S, et al. Achieving accurate ligament balancing using robotic-assisted unicompartmental knee arthroplasty. Adv Orthop 2013;2013:837167

8. Pearle AD, van der List JP, Lee L, Coon TM, Borus TA, Roche MW. Survivorship and patient satisfaction of robotic-assisted medial unicompartmental knee arthroplasty at a minimum two-year follow-up. Knee 2017;24(2):419–428

9. Batailler C, White N, Ranaldi FM, Neyret P, Servien E, Lustig S. Improved implant position and lower revision rate with robotic-assisted unicompartmental knee arthroplasty. Knee Surg Sports Traumatol Arthrosc 2019;27(4):1232–1240

10. Zhang F, Li H, Ba Z, Bo C, Li K. Robotic arm-assisted vs conventional unicompartmental knee arthroplasty: A meta-analysis of the effects on clinical outcomes. Medicine (Baltimore) 2019; 98(35):e16968

11. Blyth MJG, Anthony I, Rowe P, Banger MS, MacLean A, Jones B. Robotic arm-assisted *versus* conventional unicompartmental knee arthroplasty: Exploratory secondary analysis of a randomised controlled trial. Bone Joint Res 2017;6(11):631–639

12. van der List JP, Chawla H, Joskowicz L, Pearle AD. Current state of computer navigation and robotics in unicompartmental and total knee arthroplasty: a systematic review with meta-analysis. Knee Surg Sports Traumatol Arthrosc 2016;24(11):3482–3495

13. Waldstein W, Bou Monsef J, Buckup J, Boettner F. The value of valgus stress radiographs in the workup for medial unicompartmental arthritis. Clin Orthop Relat Res 2013;471(12):3998–4003

Handheld Robotics in Total Knee Replacement

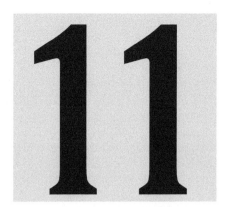

Anoop Jhurani, Mukesh Aswal, and Piyush Agarwal

Introduction

- Obtaining optimal limb alignment and soft tissue balance is the standard goal for total knee arthroplasty (TKA).[1] However, it can be difficult to achieve in every case, especially with severe coronal and/or sagittal deformity.[2]
- Robotics are designed to increase the chances of achieving this goal in every case, irrespective of the extent of deformity[2] (**Fig. 11.1**).

- The surgical procedure utilizing robotics involves the sequence shown in **Flowchart 11.1**.
- Robotic-assisted TKA has found to reduce the number of mechanical axis outliers along with improving the clinical and functional outcomes.[3]
- Benefits of robotic-assisted TKA are[4–7]:
  - Accurate bony cuts.
  - Restoration of knee kinematics and soft tissue balance.
  - Improved prosthesis survival and function.

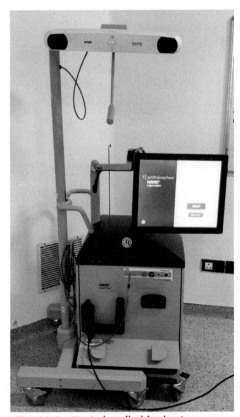

Fig. 11.1 Navio handheld robotics.

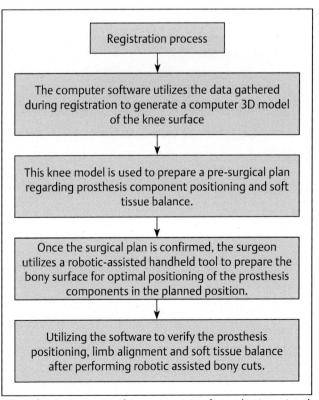

Flowchart 11.1 Working sequence for robotic-assisted surgery.

– Presurgical planning.
– Real-time interpretation and feedback of soft tissue behavior intraoperatively.
– Reduced requirement of instruments and inventory.

Instruments

• Special instruments required in robotics are (**Fig. 11.2** to **Fig. 11.6**):
  – Burrs of different shape and sizes (left to right) (**Fig. 11.4**):
    ○ Cylindrical.
    ○ 5-mm spherical.
    ○ 2-mm spherical.

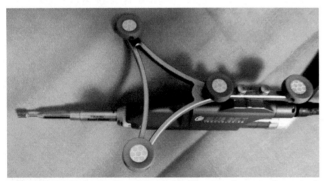

Fig. 11.2 Robotic handpiece for burring in speed control mode.

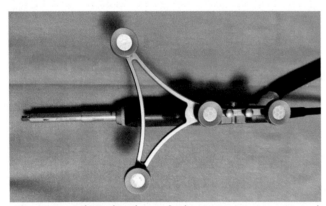

Fig. 11.3 Robotic handpiece for burring in exposure control mode.

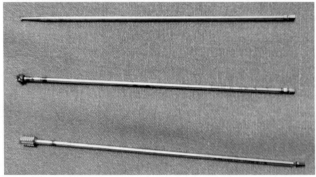

Fig. 11.4 Burrs.

– Robotic instruments (left to right) (**Fig. 11.5**):
  ○ First row: Guards, plane visualization tool, T-handle wrench, tissue protector, Z-knee retractor.
  ○ Second row: Bone pins, handpiece tracker array, femur tracker array, tibia tracker array, point probe.
  ○ Third row: Tracker array clamps.
– Pointer and arrays with flat markers (**Fig. 11.6**).
• As per the requirements during surgery, burr and control mode can be changed (**Fig. 11.7**).

Checkpoints

• A static landmark can be made as a checkpoint to verify the position of arrays during surgery.

> **Pearls**
>
> Depression over the tibial and femoral arrays can be used as checkpoints instead of inserting extra screws in the bone (**Fig. 11.8**).

Stress Range of Motion

• The orange bar represents the medial gap and the blue bar represents the lateral gap (**Fig. 11.9**).
• Y-axis represents whether there is a "laxity" or "tightness." Above the midline represents that the soft tissues are lax and below represents tightness.
• The X-axis represents the range of motion of the knee from 0 to 120 degrees.
• The vertical blue interrupted line indicates the angle at which the patient's neutral position was collected.
• Both the varus and valgus stress range of movement is collected in a TKA to assess the soft tissues.

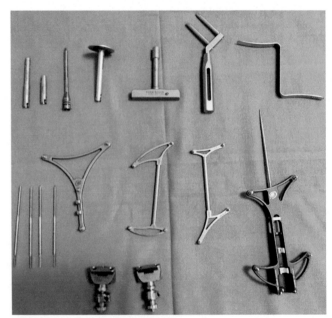

Fig. 11.5 Robotic instruments.

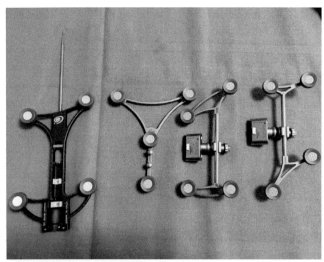

Fig. 11.6 Pointer and arrays.

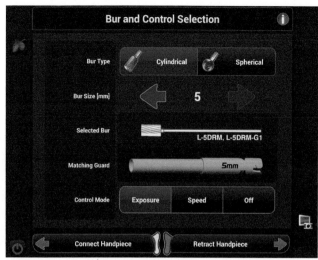

Fig. 11.7 Burr and control selection.

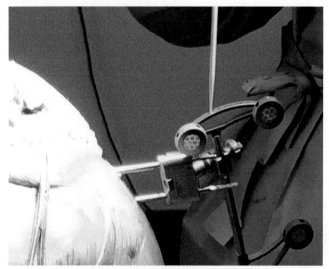

Fig. 11.8 Checkpoint marking.

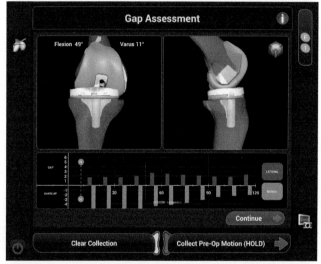

Fig. 11.9 Stress range of motion.

Pearls

Z-retractor provided in the instrument box can be used as a distracter to provide equal force in the medial and lateral compartments throughout the ROM (**Fig. 11.10**).

- It is advisable to focus on the joint space of the loose compartment with the knee in full extension. Prosthesis placement and ligament releases open up the tighter compartment.
- Adjustments to the femoral component rotation should be carefully considered. Caution needs to be exercised regarding anterior notching or overstuffing.
- Confirm that the bony resection is appropriate for the femur and tibia in extension as well as flexion.

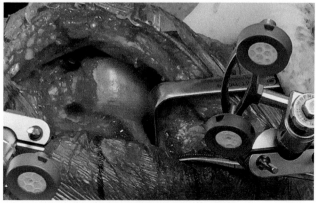

Fig. 11.10 Stress range of motion collection.

- The final gap graph should reflect an appropriate level of laxity in the joint in a tensioned state.

Component Planning

- Robotics chooses bigger size in case the femur or tibia is between 2 component sizes (**Table 11.1**).

Pearls

Cross-sectional views on robotic planning screen should be used to assess the correct size of prosthetic components.

Bone Cuts

There are three methods for removing bone from the femur:
- Femur Cut Guide:
  - A cutting guide jig is attached to the bone and an oscillating saw is used to cut the bone.
- Distal Burring:
  - It's a hybrid method for femur bone preparation with the combined use of saw and burr.
  - Initially, the distal femur is burred, followed by the attachment of AP cutting jig in the two peg holes to complete the cuts.
  - A cutting jig is attached for the tibial cut with the help of verification probe.

- Burr All Technique
  - Entire femur and tibial preparation are done by burring the bone instead of cutting with a saw.

Planning Bone Cuts

- A 3D model can be used to predict the thickness of the bony cut (**Fig. 11.11** to **Fig. 11.14**).
- Cartilage wear needs to be considered while planning the bony cuts.
- If the cartilage is worn out but bone is not eroded then additional 2 mm may be added to the resection.
- However, if bone erosion is present, then 3 mm needs to be added to the normally planned resection.
- Depending on the color of the bar joining the two condylar cuts, the distal femur cut can be predicted.

Pitfalls

It is not possible to cross-check the thickness of the bony cuts after burring.

Pearls

- The authors prefer to keep the distal femoral cut in 0.5 degree of varus and tibial cut in 1-degree varus.
- It is advised to keep the femoral component in 4-degree flexion and the tibial component in 4 degrees of posterior slope to get accurate prosthesis positioning post burring.

Table 11.1 Kinematics and its correction sequence

Scenario	Manipulation
Gap is tight in both flexion and extension	Increase the thickness of tibial cut.
Gap is tight in flexion only	Downsize the femoral component or Increase the posterior tibial slope
Balance is tight in the medial compartment in flexion	Increase external rotation of the femur component by 2 to 3 degrees to balance
Balance is tight in extension only	Increase distal femur cut
Balance is loose in extension and flexion	Decrease tibial cut thickness
Gap is loose in flexion	Upsize femoral component or Decrease tibial slope
Gap is loose in extension (recurvatum knees)	Decrease distal femur cut
Balance is loose in the medial compartment in flexion	Avoid overzealous medial release or downsizing tibia as this may further increase the medial flexion gap

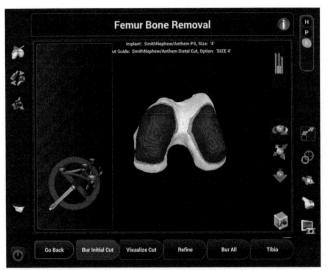

Fig. 11.11 Distal femur cut < 8.5 mm.

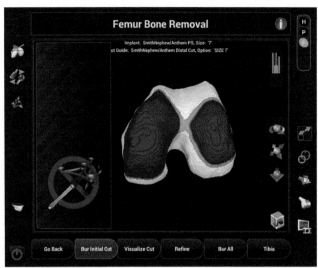

Fig. 11.12 Distal femur cut = 9 mm.

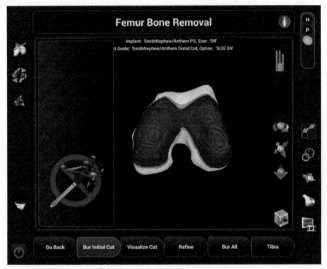

Fig. 11.13 Distal femur cut 9.5 mm.

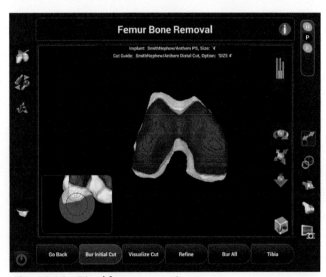

Fig. 11.14 Distal femur cut > 10 mm.

Visualizing the Cut

- This step enables the surgeon to verify the executed cut in comparison to the planned cut.
- The plane visualization tool that attaches to the handpiece is kept on the cut bony surfaces.
- This helps ensure that the rotation of the component and the depth of the bony cuts are consistent with the plan.
- The cuts can be visualized in all the three anatomic planes. In **Fig. 11.15**, counterclockwise from the upper right, these views are the sagittal, coronal, and transverse views.
- A solid line represents the cross-section of the plane visualization tool relative to the bone.
- A dotted line will appear for either the distal cut plane, anterior cut plane, or the proximal cut plane in case of the tibia.

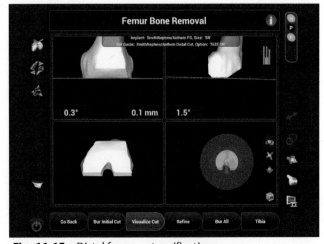

Fig. 11.15 Distal femur cut verification.

Case 1: Varus with Fixed Flexion Deformity

- Severe knee arthritis with varus deformity can be seen on clinical and radiological images (**Fig. 11.16**).
- Hip joint center is collected first with gentle hip rotation in anticlockwise direction (**Fig. 11.17**).
- Initially abduct the hip and stabilize the pelvis. Thereafter start rotating the lower limb at the hip for collecting the center of the hip joint.

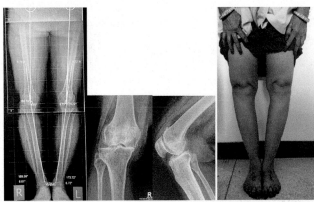

Fig. 11.16 Preoperative radiographs and image of the patient.

- As the handheld pointer paints over the bony surface, Navio creates a virtual three-dimensional model of the femur and tibia, depicting the articular bony surface (**Fig. 11.18**).
- All the osteophytes, anterior cruciate ligament (ACL), anterior synovium, and the menisci need to be removed before registration (**Fig. 11.19**).
- A right-angled Homan retractor can be placed just anterior to PCL to translate the tibia anteriorly for registration.
- The planning screen shows 9 degrees of varus and 7 degrees of flexion deformity (**Fig. 11.20**).
- The kinematic analysis demonstrates loose lateral gap throughout the ROM with a correctable medial joint gap (**Fig. 11.21**).
- The lateral gap was much more lax in comparison to the medial gap (**Fig. 11.22**).

Pitfalls

The femoral component size should be checked with manual sizer as well. Robotics shows the higher size of femur when in between sizes.

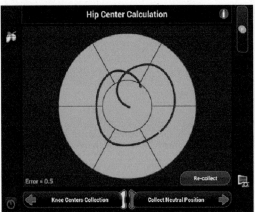

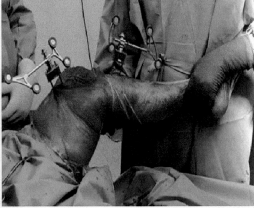

Fig. 11.17 Hip center collection.

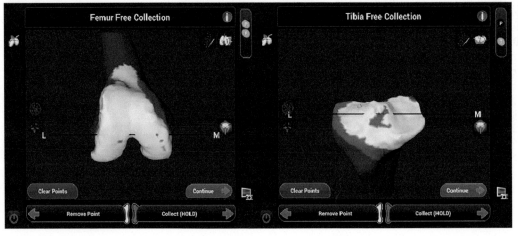

Fig. 11.18 3D model for distal femur and proximal tibia.

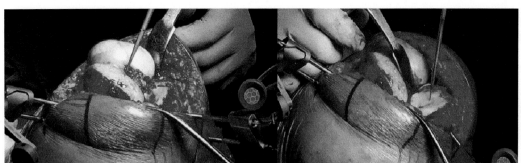

Fig. 11.19 Femur and tibia registration.

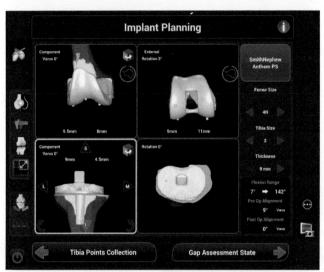

Fig. 11.20 Initial planning screen.

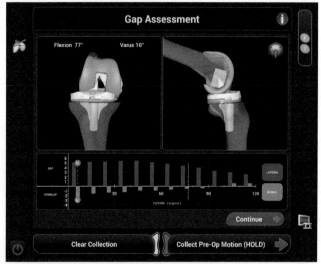

Fig. 11.21 Stress range of motion (ROM).

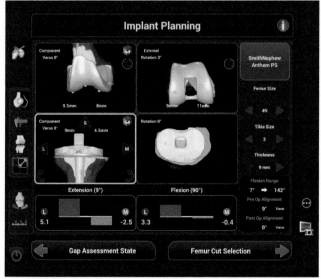

Fig. 11.22 Initial planning screen with limb alignment and gap balancing.

Pearls

The tibial slope can be altered according to the implant being used:

- CR = 5 degrees.
- PS = 3 degrees.
- 3 to 7 degrees in female patients as the natural slope is comparatively more.
- 0 to 3 degrees in PS knee with severe FFD to close the flexion gap.

- The distal femur cut and the proximal tibia cut were decreased by 1 mm (**Fig. 11.23**).
- The residual tightness of the medial side was corrected by posteromedial release.
- The thickness of the bony cut is color coded (**Fig. 11.24**).
    - Purple denotes > 5 mm.
    - Blue denotes 3 to 4 mm.
    - Green denotes 1 to 2 mm.
    - Pink represents 1 mm overcut.
    - Red represents >2 mm depression.

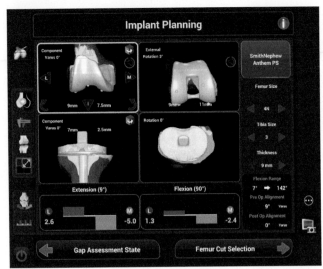

Fig. 11.23 Final planning with gap balancing.

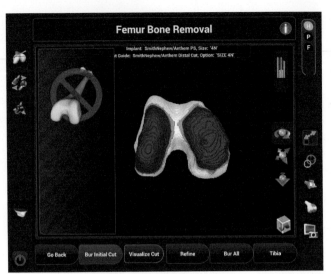

Fig. 11.24 Initial distal femur burr.

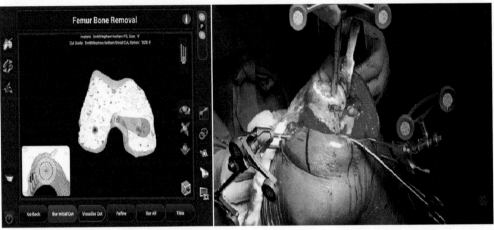

Fig. 11.25 Burring distal femur.

- Excessive pressure over the burr could create punch holes in case of osteoporotic bone.
- The surgeon can predict the thickness of the distal femur cut from this screen.
- If both the femoral condyle cuts are connected with a blue bar, the cut is around 10 mm.
- The distal femur was burred as per the plan (**Fig. 11.25**).
- Care is to be exerted to cause minimal red punch zones.
- Accuracy of bony cuts can be checked with plane verification tool. the goal is to achieve the accuracy of bony cuts within 1 degree of the plan (**Fig. 11.26**).
- Clinical and robotic screen showing tibial all-burr technique with verification (**Fig. 11.27** and **Fig. 11.28**).

- Postoperative ROM and final alignment with correction of the deformity can be seen on postoperative screen (**Fig. 11.29**).
- The postoperative gap assessment screen shows 1- to 2-mm of opening which is desirable for a smooth range of movement of the knee (**Fig. 11.30**).
- Final assessment screen for preoperative and the postoperative limb alignment. The femoral and tibial components with insert are shown in **Fig. 11.31**.
- The postoperative X-Ray shows well-aligned components (**Fig. 11.32**).

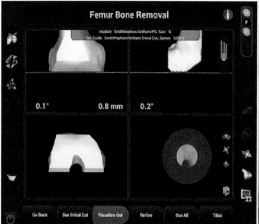

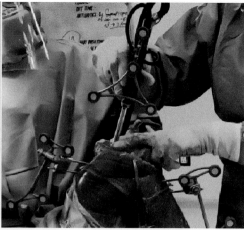

Fig. 11.26 Distal femur burr verification.

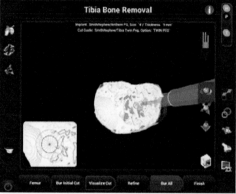

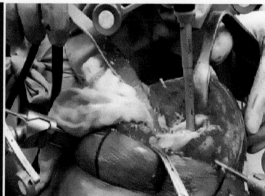

Fig. 11.27 Burring of proximal tibia.

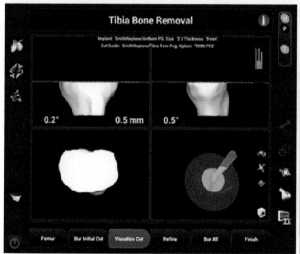

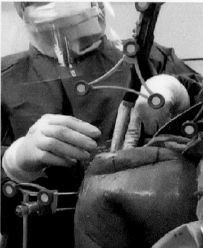

Fig. 11.28 Proximal tibia burr verification.

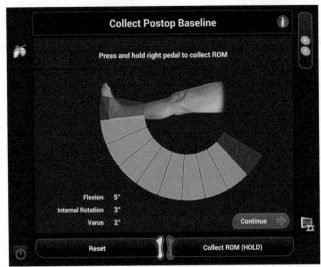

Fig. 11.29 Baseline range of motion (ROM).

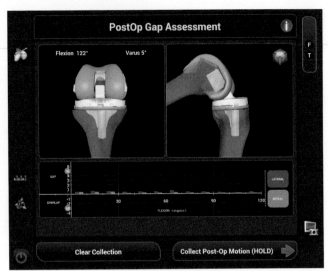

Fig. 11.30 Postoperative gap assessment.

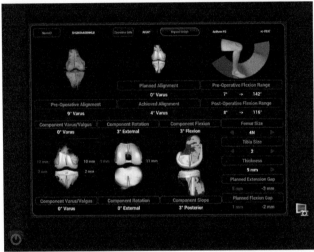

Fig. 11.31 Final report.

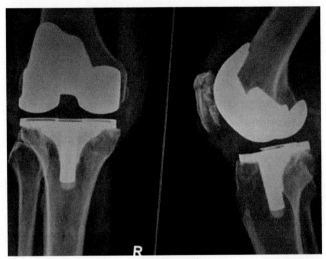

Fig. 11.32 Postoperative radiographs.

Case 2: Valgus with Flexion Deformity

- Clinical and radiological image demonstrates a windswept deformity with valgus deformity of right knee (**Fig. 11.33**).
- The external rotation of the femoral component needs to be increased in valgus deformities to compensate lateral femoral condyle hypoplasia (**Fig. 11.34** and **Fig.11.35**).
- The preoperative gap assessment shows tight lateral gaps in extension and a loose medial gap in flexion (**Fig. 11.36**).
- The preplanning screen demonstrates 4 degrees of valgus with 5 degrees of flexion (**Fig. 11.37**).
- An increased distal femoral cut was planned to compensate for the loose flexion gap (**Fig. 11.38**).

- The tight lateral gap in extension warranted IT band pie crusting to balance the knee.
- Image showing all-burr technique for femur and tibia (**Fig. 11.39**).
- A well-seated trial prosthesis after all-burr femur (**Fig. 11.40**).
- The residual tight lateral flexion gap was balanced by pie crusting of the popliteus tendon and IT band for extension (**Fig. 11.41** and **Fig. 11.42**).
- The postoperative gap assessment shows 1- to 2-mm joint opening throughout the ROM (**Fig. 11.43**).
- A well-balanced knee with well aligned prosthesis is seen on postoperative radiographs (**Fig. 11.44**).

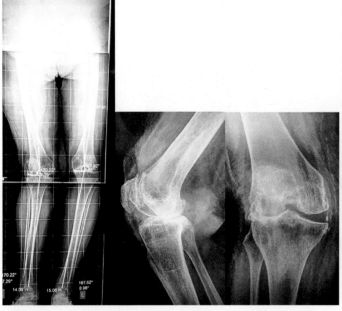
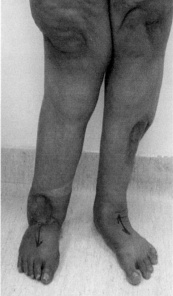

Fig. 11.33 Preoperative radiographs and image of the patient.

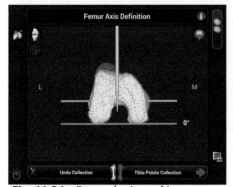

Fig. 11.34 Femoral axis marking.

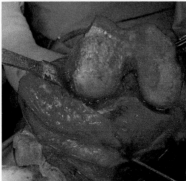

Fig. 11.35 Lateral condyle hypoplasia.

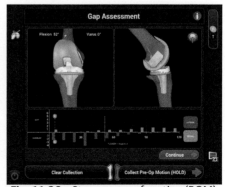

Fig. 11.36 Stress range of motion (ROM).

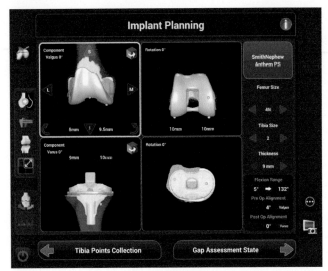

Fig. 11.37 Initial planning screen.

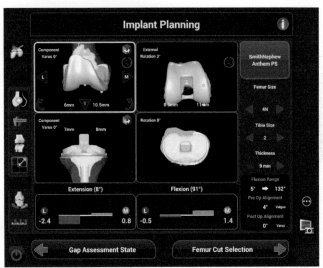

Fig. 11.38 Final planning and gap balancing.

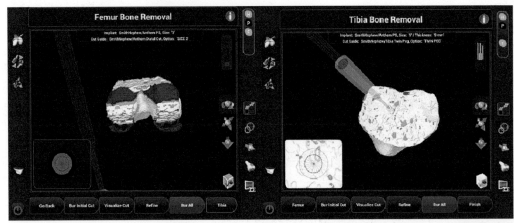

Fig. 11.39 All-burr femur and tibia.

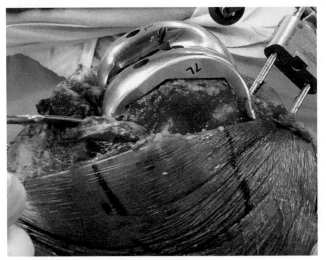

Fig. 11.40 Well-seated femur trial.

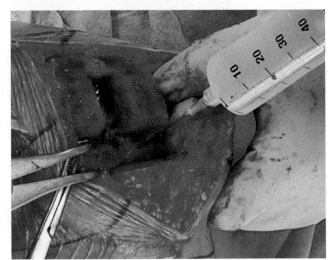

Fig. 11.41 Popliteus tendon pie crusting.

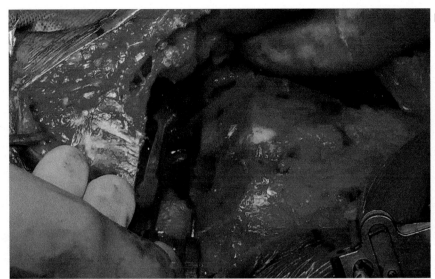

Fig. 11.42 Iliotibial (IT) band pie crusting.

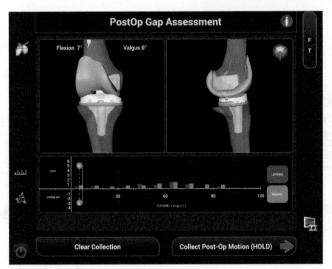

Fig. 11.43 Postoperative gap assessment.

Fig. 11.44 Postoperative radiographs.

Case 3: Severe Varus Deformity

- The preoperative radiographs and clinical image demonstrate a subluxed knee with a wide lateral joint space opening (**Fig. 11.45**).
- The preoperative robotic screen shows a 23 degrees varus with neutral sagittal alignment (**Fig. 11.46**).
- Robotic screen showing gap balance before and after bone cuts and implant planning (**Fig. 11.47**).
- The aim of planning is to bring the violet bar (lateral gap) above the midline representing 1- to 2-mm of opening.
- One should not aim to bring the orange bar (medial gap) above the midline as it represents the tight medial gap which can only be corrected by soft tissue releases and not by component adjustment.
- The external rotation of the femoral component was increased to balance the tight medial and the loose lateral gap in flexion.

- The distal femoral cut was reduced to 8 mm because correction of the severe varus deformity results in an increased extension gap.
- The residual tight medial gap required posteromedial soft tissue release and reduction osteotomy of tibia.
- Robotic screen showing distal femur and proximal tibia bone surface post burring (**Fig. 11.48** and **Fig. 11.49**).
- With trial components, the knee was tight in both flexion and extension with persisting lateral laxity.
- To compensate for the residual medial tightness, downsizing of the tibial component was done.
- An additional 1 mm of the proximal cut was taken in 1 degree of varus to increase the medial gap in comparison to the lateral gap (**Fig. 11.50**).
- Such fine adjustments in the tibial slope and coronal plane alignment are possible only with the help of robotic-assisted surgery.

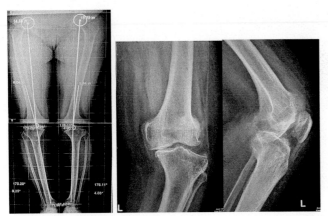

Fig. 11.45 Preoperative radiographs.

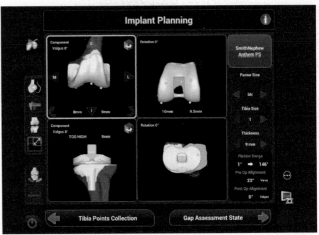

Fig. 11.46 Initial planning screen.

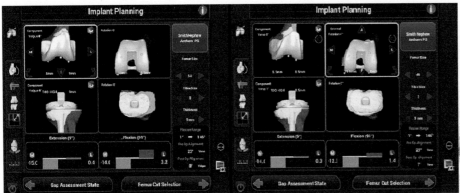

Fig. 11.47 Final planning screen after gap balancing.

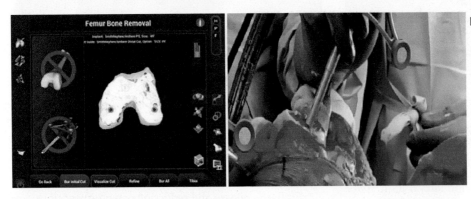

Fig. 11.48 Distal femur burr.

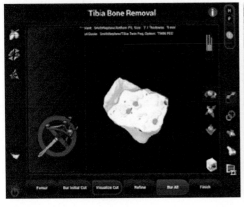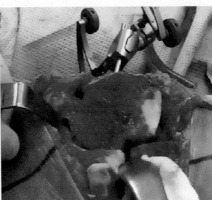

Fig. 11.49 Proximal tibia burr.

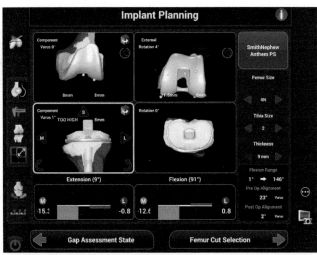

Fig. 11.50 Replanning after trial.

- The posteromedial soft tissues were released and medial osteophytes were removed to balance the mediolateral gap (**Fig. 11.51**).
- The postoperative ROM show complete correction of the coronal plane deformity with mediolaterally balanced knee throughout arc of motion (**Fig. 11.52**).
- Well-aligned and balanced knee seen in postoperative radiographs (**Fig. 11.53**).

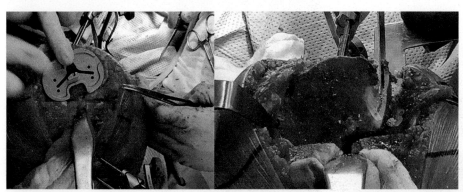

Fig. 11.51 Posteromedial reduction osteotomy to correct tight medial gap.

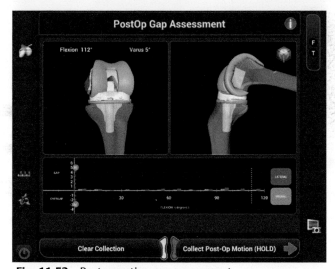

Fig. 11.52 Postoperative gap assessment.

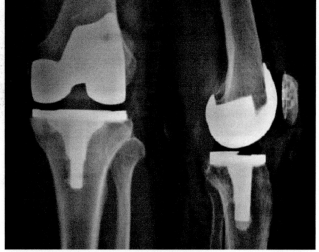

Fig. 11.53 Postoperative radiographs.

Case 4: Varus with Recurvatum Deformity

- Severe tibiofemoral arthritis with varus-recurvatum deformity can be seen on clinical and radiological images (**Fig. 11.54**).
- The implant planning screen shows 11 degrees of varus and 2 degrees of recurvatum deformity (**Fig. 11.55**).
- Each knee has unique kinematic pattern which changes with knee flexion.

- Conventional knee radiographs and clinical examination with the knee in extension only reveal lateral joint laxity and tightness of the medial structures.
- Robotics gives additional information about soft tissue behavior in knee flexion.
- The kinematic analysis demonstrates loose lateral gap throughout the ROM with a correctable tight medial joint gap (**Fig. 11.56**).
- An image suggestive of anterior femoral notching. The lateral, femoral, cross-section views should be checked to identify the femur component position (**Fig. 11.57**).
- The femoral component should be sitting flush with the anterior femoral cortex to maintain the anterior offset.
- The preplanning screen showing loose lateral and tight medial gap (**Fig. 11.58**).

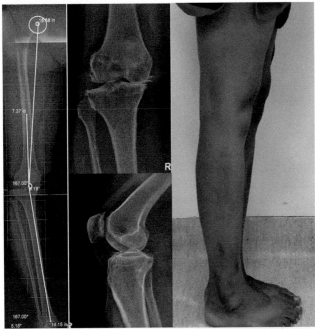

Fig. 11.54 Preoperative radiographs and clinical image of the patient.

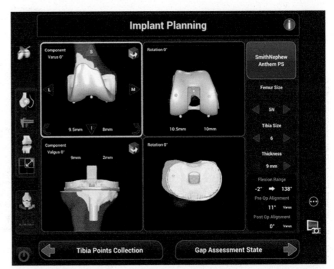

Fig. 11.55 Implant planning screen.

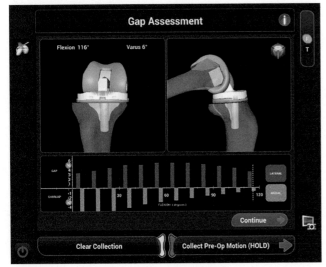

Fig. 11.56 Stress range of motion (ROM).

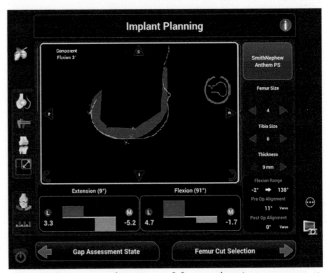

Fig. 11.57 Coronal section of femur showing component flush with anterior cortex.

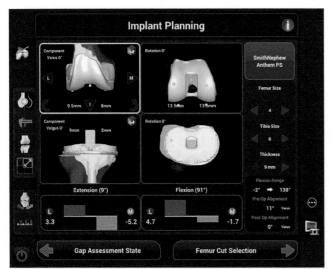

Fig. 11.58 Initial alignment and gap balancing.

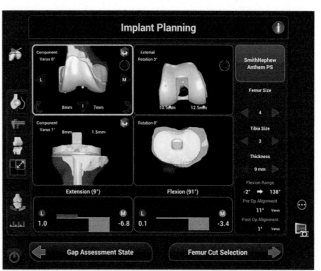

Fig. 11.59 Planned cuts and alignment.

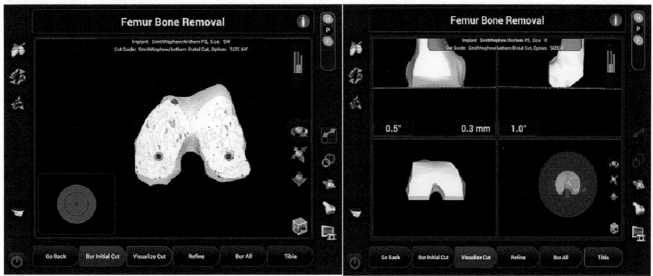

Fig. 11.60 Distal femur burr and verification.

- The distal femur cut and the proximal tibia cut were decreased by 2 mm (**Fig. 11.59**).
- The residual tightness of the medial side was corrected by posteromedial release.
- The distal femur was burred as per the plan and cuts verified (**Fig. 11.60**).
- Similarly, tibia was burred with all-burr technique (**Fig. 11.61**).

- Final alignment of 5 degrees flexion with complete correction of coronal deformity can be seen on postoperative screen (**Fig. 11.62**).
- Final assessment screen for preoperative and postoperative limb alignment (**Fig. 11.63**).
- The postoperative X-ray shows well-aligned components (**Fig. 11.64**).

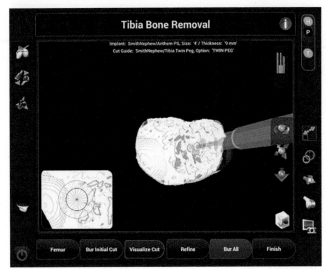

Fig. 11.61 Proximal tibia burr.

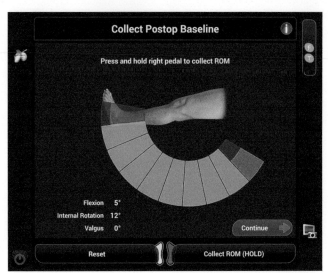

Fig. 11.62 Baseline range of motion (ROM) with final alignment.

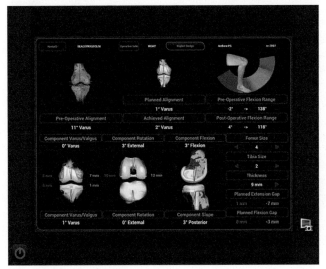

Fig. 11.63 Final report.

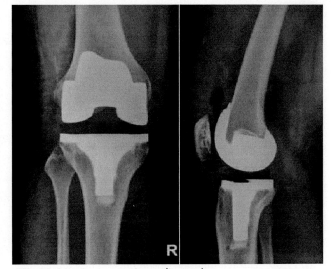

Fig. 11.64 Postoperative radiographs.

Points to Remember

- In robotic-assisted surgery, it is not possible to measure the distal femur cut. Hence, attention should be paid to the distal femur burr screen.
- For standard cut, the two condyles should be joined by blue or violet (2–3 mm).
- The aim of gap planning in a varus knee is to get violet bar (lateral gap) above the midline showing 1- to 2-mm opening in lateral joint space. this can be done by adjusting the thickness of the cut and implant position.
- The orange bar representing tight medial gap will be corrected only by soft tissue releases.
- For a valgus knee, the orange bar (medial side) can be adjusted just above the midline by thickness of the cut and implant position.
- The tight lateral side (violet bar) will come above the midline only after lateral soft tissue releases.
- Handheld robotics has a learning curves as a surgeon needs to adapt to the burring technique instead of using a conventional saw. it is recommended that the surgeon should first practice doing distal femur burr before graduating to the all burr femur technique.

References

1. Gromov K, Korchi M, Thomsen MG, Husted H, Troelsen A. What is the optimal alignment of the tibial and femoral components in knee arthroplasty? Acta Orthop 2014;85(5):480–487

2. Marchand RC, Sodhi N, Khlopas A, et al. Coronal correction for severe deformity using robotic-assisted total knee arthroplasty. J Knee Surg 2018;31(1):2–5

3. Song EK, Seon JK, Yim JH, Netravali NA, Bargar WL. Robotic-assisted TKA reduces postoperative alignment outliers and improves gap balance compared to conventional TKA. [published correction appears in Clin Orthop Relat Res. 2012 Sep;470(9):2627] Clin Orthop Relat Res 2013;471(1):118–126

4. Lonner JH, Fillingham YA. Pros and cons: a balanced view of robotics in knee arthroplasty. J Arthroplasty 2018;33(7):2007–2013

5. Mancuso F, Pandit H. Robotics accuracy in orthopaedics: is it enough for a well-working knee replacement? Ann Transl Med 2016;4(Suppl 1):S39

6. Moon YW, Ha CW, Do KH, et al. Comparison of robot-assisted and conventional total knee arthroplasty: a controlled cadaver study using multiparameter quantitative three-dimensional CT assessment of alignment. Comput Aided Surg 2012;17(2):86–95

7. Clark TC, Schmidt FH. Robot-assisted navigation versus computer-assisted navigation in primary total knee arthroplasty: efficiency and accuracy. ISRN Orthop 2013;2013:794827

Index